P9-BZI-091

Robert A. Harrell, M.D.
Attending Physician
Durham County General Hospital
Consulting Associate
Department of Medicine
Duke University School of Medicine
Durham, North Carolina

Gary S. Firestein, M.D.
Assistant Professor
Department of Medicine
University of California
San Diego, California

With an Introduction by
Philip A. Tumulty, M.D.
David J. Carver Professor Emeritus of Medicine
Johns Hopkins University School of Medicine
Baltimore, Maryland

And Contributions by
Mark W. Woodruff, M.D.
Duke-Watts Family Medicine Program
Durham, North Carolina

APPLETON & LANGE
Norwalk, Connecticut/San Mateo, California

0-8385-2120-7

Notice: Our knowledge in clinical sciences is constantly changing. As new information becomes available, changes in treatment and in the use of drugs become necessary. The author(s) and the publisher of this volume have taken care to make certain that the doses of drugs and schedules of treatment are correct and compatible with the standards generally accepted at the time of publication. The reader is advised to consult carefully the instruction and information material included in the package insert of each drug or therapeutic agent before administration. This advice is especially important when using new or infrequently used drugs.

Copyright © 1988 by Appleton & Lange
A Publishing Division of Prentice Hall
Copyright © 1981, 1983 by Arco Publishing, Inc.

All rights reserved. This book, or any parts thereof, may not be used or reproduced in any manner without written permission. For information, address Appleton & Lange, 25 Van Zant Street, East Norwalk, Connecticut 06855.

88 89 90 91 92 / 10 9 8 7 6 5 4 3 2 1

Prentice-Hall International (UK) Limited, *London*
Prentice-Hall of Australia Pty. Limited, *Sydney*
Prentice-Hall Canada, Inc., *Toronto*
Prentice-Hall Hispanoamericana, S.A., *Mexico*
Prentice-Hall of India Private Limited, *New Delhi*
Prentice-Hall of Japan, Inc., *Tokyo*
Simon & Schuster Asia Pte. Ltd., *Singapore*
Editora Prentice-Hall do Brasil Ltda., *Rio de Janeiro*
Prentice-Hall, *Englewood Cliffs, New Jersey*

Library of Congress Cataloging-in-Publication Data
Harrell, Robert A.
  The effective scutboy/Robert A. Harrell, Gary S. Firestein;
with an introduction by Philip Tumulty; and contributions by Mark
W. Woodruff. – 3rd ed.
    p.   cm.
  ISBN 0-8385-2120-7
  1. Medicine, Clinical–Study and teaching. 2. Medical students.
3. Medicine, Clinical–Handbooks, manuals, etc. I. Firestein, Gary
S. II. Woodruff, Mark W. III. Title.
  [DNLM: 1. Education, Medical. 2. Medicine–handbooks.
3. Students, Medical. W 18 H296e]
R834.H34 1988
616'.0073–dc19
DNLM/DLC   88-10472
for Library of Congress   CIP

Acquisitions Editor: R. Craig Percy
Production Editor: Elizabeth C. Ryan
Designer: Steven M. Byrum

PRINTED IN THE UNITED STATES OF AMERICA

THE EFFECTIVE SCUTBOY

The Principles and Practice of Scut

3RD Edition

THE EFFECTIVE
SCUTBOY

The Principles and Practice of Scut

3RD Edition

W
⅋
+296₽
988

⟩

Contents

3 0001 00326 1734

17804257

Preface

It is hard to believe that nearly a decade has passed since the origin of *The Effective Scutboy*. Because of a need for better transition from basic sciences to clinical rotations, several talks were given on this subject in early 1979 at the Pithotomy Club, the Johns Hopkins medical student's eating club. Notes from these talks were typed and were given the title, *The Effective Scutboy*. These notes became widely distributed at Johns Hopkins. The positive response led the authors in the summer of 1979 to expand the book into a pocket-sized manual. An initial printing of 400 was made in the fall of 1979 and sold out in a few days. A larger printing was distributed to medical bookstores across the country later that year resulting in sales of over 2000 copies of the "small grey edition." With approaching internships, we decided to find a commercial publisher to take over publication and distribution of the book. A revised edition was prepared and released by Arco Publishing Company in 1981, followed by a revised second edition in 1983. We are now pleased to have Appleton & Lange publishing the third edition.

Since the original publication of *The Effective Scutboy*, several books have attempted to encompass some of our goals. However, we believe that this book remains the only publication devoted exclusively to providing practical information for medical students in the difficult transition from basic sciences to clinical rotations. For this edition, we are continuing to broaden the applicability of the book to all medical schools as well as related fields, such as nursing and physician's assistant programs. New features in this edition include sections on pediatrics,

OB-GYN, and surgery rotations, and greater emphasis on special types of notes, outpatient settings, prescriptions, and understanding the role of all health professionals.

We would like to thank R. Craig Percy and Elizabeth C. Ryan of Appleton & Lange for their support and help. We remain grateful to Dr. Philip Tumulty for his timeless introduction and his inspiration to us as an effective clinician.

Robert A. Harrell, M.D.
Durham, North Carolina

Gary S. Firestein, M.D.
San Diego, California

Introduction

This book presents very succinctly and accurately how the practical requirements of being an effective clinical clerk can best be met. We would like to add to these essentials a brief discussion of some of the more philosophical aspects of an effective clerkship.

Clearly, the purpose of a clinical clerkship is to become familiar with the responsibilities, approaches, and techniques, as well as the attributes, of an accomplished clinician. Needless to say, this is a very large order, and in the usual eight-week clerkship only a beginning can be made. It must be a beginning that provides a fast start and encompasses what clinical medicine is really all about and, believe me, what it is actually all about is not nearly so much techniques and methods as it is personal attributes and a proper approach to sick persons and their problems.

But let's get down to particulars. A patient lies in front of you on a bed. As a clinical clerk it is essential that you regard yourself as a genuine member of the team sharing the heavy personal responsibilities for the care of this sick person, and that you not perceive yourself to be merely a clerk, technician, messenger, or some kind of *agent provocateur* standing at the periphery of the medical action. If you have the ability, the interest, and personal concern, your impact upon the welfare of this patient will go far beyond "scut" work—although, to be sure, in all of its phases and for all of us, regardless of age or status, clinical medicine necessarily imposes a diet of milk as well as cream and, generally, a lot more of the former than the latter.

You can be absolutely certain of one thing: Regardless of

intellectual, emotional, or social status, this patient will reach out to you and hold on to you as his or her physician, not in relationship to your age, experience, rank, or status, but rather in accordance with the genuineness of your interest. The patient will judge you by the degree to which you help, comfort, and support in small, but very human, ways, as well as in the big "decision making."

Whether or not you are accepted warmly by your assigned patients as their "young physician" depends entirely upon whether or not you understand what the role of a clinician really is and attempt to play it to the fullest of your intellectual, physical, and emotional capacities. Clinical experience and knowledge come only with time—much time. An intense, active desire to serve and give of yourself to sick persons is immediate in its development, and any clinical clerk having this desire doesn't need to fret about personal status on the wards. To your patients you will be an exceedingly important, effective, and indispensable individual. As we have already indicated, this will be true whether the patient is rich or poor, black or white, old or young, organically ill or emotionally disturbed, highly intelligent or intellectually deprived. The response to genuine caring is universal.

In order to care for someone adequately, it is of course essential that one learns how to effectively communicate with that person. This, in turn, depends upon a general knowledge of and familiarity with the broad range of frequently highly complex aspects of human nature. A frequent complaint of so many patients today is the failure of their physician to communicate with them in a meaningful fashion. How unfortunate—for clearly, to help this sick patient lying before you, you must accomplish certain things and do them well.

First, you must obtain an accurate and meticulously complete history of the patient's illness. This involves not only a recitation of the cold facts of the illness, but also an understanding and appreciation of the patient who is ill, including personal characteristics and family and social setting.

Second, you must be able to have a strong, positive impact on the patient so that you can provide the guidance, support, and insight that all sick persons must have if they are to handle their illnesses in an effective and positive manner. You will be asking and expecting your patients to do many things that are exceedingly hard for people to do, from losing twenty-five pounds to having a lung removed. Unless you have the capacity to impel your patients by the strength of the personal impact you have on them, you cannot possibly anticipate or expect a really satisfying therapeutic result.

Third, you must have the same sort of positive impact on involved family members. Sickness in a husband, wife, or parent is always a family affair, and you must not isolate yourself from the family. They will need the same guidance, advice, and support that you give to the patient; otherwise, your care of the patient will quickly become an empty effort.

It is obvious that these three essential functions of an effective clinician have as a common denominator the ability to communicate effectively with all kinds of people, in all sorts of life circumstances.

Therefore, as a clinical clerk, make one of your major goals the acquisition of familiarity with the reactions of human nature as they present themselves in a host of guises and circumstances. Learn to work with human nature, how to relate to it, how to influence it, in a way that is positively impelling.

How can this be accomplished when you are just starting out as a clerk? By spending adequate time sitting at the bedside and listening to your patients each day as they "unload" their questions, concerns, and problems. Give any of your patients the opportunity and they will tell you their life stories. Through such revelations comes a growing understanding of the "inner person." Do the same thing with concerned relatives. For example, what concerns and emotions dominate the mind of a 47-year-old father of three young children who gets a "precordial pain" while working as a laborer at a local steel plant? Or again, what is the impact of the presence of a malignant disease on any human being? Through your ability to communicate, how can you supplant negative reactions and emotions with positive ones and thus relieve human suffering, bringing about at the very least an improvement in emotional health? This is what clinical medicine is really all about. An excellent clinician, therefore, is not so much a clever "doer" as he is an effective communicator, and the acquisition of this invaluable ability must start from your very first day on the wards.

It sounds trite to stress the necessity of being expert in all aspects of the physical examination of the sick person lying before you. Nevertheless, experience proves that even in this day of fantastic technical diagnostic achievement, the primacy of the physical examination remains untouched. So make it a point during your clerkship to have as many clinical experiences as you possibly can. Take every opportunity to observe some clinical finding not familiar to you before, so that your experience in physical diagnosis becomes as broad and sophisticated as you can possibly make it. A very "routine" admission oftentimes will contain new learning experiences if you only look, find, and observe.

In this regard, let me make a lamentation that I feel very keenly: The parochial attitude that so many clinical clerks have vastly inhibits their learning opportunities. By this I mean that while some students may faithfully "work up" assigned patients, they will make no effort to extend their observations to other patients. Thus, a patient on Ward 5 may have an intense pericardial friction rub, but you won't go and listen to it and learn because you are assigned to Ward 4. Realize that the entire patient population of the medical service is your "textbook of clinical medicine"—be aggressive in searching for new learning experiences. Don't cheat yourself by lazy or blasé parochialism!

In addition to being able to communicate and examine effectively, the clinician is also one who soundly manages the illnesses of his patients, both diagnostically and therapeutically. Therefore, a clinician is not so much a technical doer as a thinker and planner, the coordinator and the conductor of the medical team.

This role cannot be accomplished in a helter-skelter, off-the-cuff, moment-to-moment fashion. It requires the preparation and continuous revision of a *flow sheet*, which in a step-by-step, progressive fashion outlines in detail the diagnostic and therapeutic measures that must be taken to secure an optimum solution to the patient's health problems. These flow sheets must be reviewed and updated every day as new information is collected and changes in each patient's status occur. Such flow sheets must always be subject to the critical analysis of the entire medical team caring for the patient, including the student clerk. Such work sheets must be concerned with the needs of the "total" patient (social, financial, spiritual, family, community) as well as his medical requirements, for it is a human being you are planning for and not a disease state. Once again, that is what clinical medicine is all about.

In preparing such a flow sheet (and in this, you, the clinical clerk, will be playing a significant role) the following questions should be foremost in your thoughts:

1. How safe is this procedure?
2. Is it really necessary?
3. Will it give essential information or just add clinical data for the chart?
4. Is there a cheaper way to get the same information?
5. How stressful for the patient will it be?
6. Does the patient understand what we are trying to accomplish with this measure?
7. Should I get a more experienced consulting opinion before doing this?
8. Are the present circumstances optimal for the accomplishment of this particular measure?

Finally, a clinician must have a sound basic knowledge of the natural history of the common diseases as they affect the various organ systems. It is to the acquisition of such fundamental information that you should be devoting your time and efforts during your clerkship, and not to the reading of the latest reports in, let us say, the *Journal of Clinical Investigation.*

How can you best accomplish this? Remember that during your clinical clerkship you will only be initiating what, it is hoped, will become a lifelong habit. Your approach must not be indiscriminate reading of various texts and journals. Information so acquired is poorly digested and quickly forgotten. Do not spend your time just "reading in the library"! Rather, spend most of your time on the wards gaining as much clinical exposure as you possibly can. Have new clinical experiences—*then* go and read about them! "I have clinical experiences first and *then* I read about them" should be your golden rule. For then what you read will have a significant, adhesive force and will stay with you. Step by step, you will build your knowledge of the natural course of diseases by experiencing them first and reading about them next.

What should you read? Obviously, there will always be practical limitations to the time you will have for reading so you need to have a system. We recommend that as soon as you have had a new clinical experience, quickly read a brief description and discussion of it in one of the standard textbooks of medicine. Later, when you have more time, read a review article that is based upon a careful analysis of the natural history of the matter in question (for example, "A Review of a Hundred Cases of Giant Cell Arteritis"). Articles dealing with "the natural history of . . ." should be the level of your reading for the next several years.

Lastly, the most routine patient in the world can be a textbook of learning for you if you are smart enough to recognize that fact and react accordingly. Example: An old man with long-standing hypertension is admitted to your service following a clear-cut left-sided hemiplegia secondary to a stroke. It all seems so obvious and so routine—what is to be learned here?

Plenty! A meticulous physical examination reveals, in addition to the hypertension, arteriosclerosis, and hemiplegia, the following:

1. Arcus senilis
2. Xanthomatous deposits about the eyes
3. Loud bruits over the carotid arteries
4. Bilateral Dupuytren's contractures
5. Heberden's nodes
6. Severe osteoarthritis
7. Bilateral varicoceles
8. An inguinal hernia
9. A very enlarged prostate
10. Severe varicose veins

Ask yourself how familiar you are with each of these items in terms of the natural history of their development and course. All of a sudden, a very routine admission becomes a veritable textbook of medicine. Once again, as so often happens in clinical medicine, what initially may be regarded as routine "scut" work becomes a rewarding learning experience if we just have the maturity, initiative, wisdom, and imagination to make it so.

Philip A. Tumulty, M.D.

SECTION 1
The Principles of Scut

A. OVERVIEW

1. *The role of the student:* Most student rotations are oriented around a hospital inpatient service. Here the role of the student is ill-defined. The approach found most useful by many medical students is to try to be the intern for your patients. Be aggressive. Try to do everything that needs to be done for your patients. However, you are better off than the intern because you have time to read and leisurely review your patients and their charts.

   You will have patients assigned to you by your resident as they are admitted. On most medical services the student does a complete admission work-up on one patient each admitting day and then follows that patient closely throughout the hospitalization. On some services, especially surgery, the student is expected to be part of a ward team managing a number of patients.

Your resident should explain exactly what is expected of you. Ask for this explanation if it is not offered.

When you are assigned specific patients, your responsibilities include:
   a. Performing and writing a complete admission work-up
   b. Doing all scut on your patient
   c. Writing all progress notes (daily)

   d. Writing all orders (when possible)

   e. Presenting your patients at morning rounds

   f. Trying to direct diagnosis and therapy as much as you can, at the very minimum, take an active role in decision making

   g. Being familiar with the diagnoses being considered for your patients and all diagnostic studies ordered or performed on them

In order to fulfill these responsibilities you *must* know what is going on with your patients. This requires cooperation between you and each patient's intern (who is responsible for the daily care of the patient). If you conscientiously do the things listed above, including scut, the interns will be impressed with your enthusiasm and interest and will take time to discuss your patients with you.

2. Members of a typical medical service

   a. Students

   b. *Interns:* Their only responsibility is patient care (any teaching they do is a favor to you). Interns are hopelessly overworked and therefore tend to be rather moody. You can provide them with a lot of help by your labor and ideas. Do not be intimidated by the interns. They are only a couple of years ahead of you

   c. *Residents:* They are responsible for teaching students as well as supervising the interns. The resident is your major resource for both direction and teaching. The quality of your resident will have a major effect on the quality of your entire experience

---

At most hospitals residents are referred to as JARs (junior assistant residents) and SARs (senior assistant residents). This terminology dates back to the early days of the Johns Hopkins Hospital where the "resident physician" had a role similar to today's "chief resident." The house staff below that level were therefore assistant residents.

---

d. *Attending physician:* This term is confusing. Although attendings are always members of the senior staff (faculty level), the term may apply to either a patient's own physician or to the attending who supervises teaching rounds with or without any formal responsibility for patient care. Many services have both of these types of attendings. Attending rounds, or teaching rounds, are usually held several times each week and consist of formal case presentations (often by the students), followed by detailed discussions of the patients. Reading about the medical conditions of your patients before these rounds will obviously make you look sharper. Realize that attendings often have a far greater input into student grades than their knowledge of a particular student might justify. If you are shy, make a special effort to speak up. We have seen excellent students receive poor grades because they were too quiet and the attending "was not impressed" by them. On the other hand try to avoid being loud and obnoxious, a common mistake. In addition to this "teaching attending," you will likely have contact with a patient's own private attending ("private slick"). Be sensitive to his or her wishes because if they are not followed some attendings can get quite upset. These attendings can teach you a lot, especially if you show an interest in their specialty

3. Other people with whom you will interact
   a. *Consultants:* Often a patient will require the expertise of or a procedure from a specialist. The specialist is consulted and gives advice to the patient's primary physicians. Usually consultants follow the patient and continue to give advice and make comments on the patient's progress.

Medical students can spend elective time on consult services acting as part of a consulting team and obtain in-depth knowledge of a particular specialty.

b. *Fellows:* Fellows are physicians who have completed training in their specialty (e.g., internal medicine) and are getting advanced training (fellowship) in a sub-specialty (e.g., cardiology). Most fellowships are of 2 or 3 years' duration and consist of both clinical and research responsibilities. You will commonly encounter clinical fellows acting as consultants.

c. *Nurses:* Make an effort to show nurses consideration and respect. They work very hard for low wages and often have a lot of practical experience from which you can benefit. Nurses will do a lot to help you if you ask nicely.

d. *Ward secretaries:* These people are responsible for taking orders off of charts, scheduling procedures and lab tests, calling consultants, and various other duties. Quality is extremely variable. Do not trust anything important to a ward secretary. Make a habit of calling consultants and scheduling important studies yourself.

e. *Laboratory technicians, x-ray technicians, phlebotomists, IV technicians, physical therapists, respiratory therapists, social workers, dietitians:* Most hospitals have many people involved in the care of your patients. They are all working under the physician's orders. Therefore, you really need to understand what these people do, and why, in order to optimally use their skills. Talk to them. Avoid the temptation to let the IV team start all of the IVs and the phlebotomy team perform all the blood drawing. Now is the time to become competent in these skills. Remember, when you are the intern they will come to you when they cannot get an IV started.

4. *Daily routine:* The daily routine begins with morning "work" rounds. It is wise to arrive early enough to talk with and examine your patients and find out what has happened to them during the night. At morning rounds you are

expected to give a two- to three-sentence summary of the progress each of your patients is making. You will also give a formal presentation (see "Presenting Cases," Part G in this section) of any new patients at this time. The rest of the day is spent running scut, working up new patients, attending lectures, conferences, and so forth.

Try to stay on the ward as much a possible. Remember that medicine is not a spectator sport. Conferences are nice, but if you are to learn how to care for patients, you must spend time around them. As Sir William Osler put it, "Do not waste the hours of daylight in listening to that which may be read at night."

With regard to being on call, there are three basic states:

a. *"Off"*: Go home when you finish your work (usually 5 to 7 P.M.).

b. *"On short"*: Pick up a new patient; do not run scut on other people's patients; go home after you have worked up the new patient (usually 7 P.M. to midnight).

c. *"On long"*: Pick up a new patient; help the intern on call run the scut on the floor; generally spend the night at the hospital; go to bed usually at midnight to 2 A.M., but you may be called back. If you stay up all night you are probably doing something wrong.

On-call schedules vary among medical schools. Once again, bear in mind that learning is best achieved when oriented around your patients. Read about what your patients have! Don't be afraid to ask questions.

B. THE WORK-UP

The patient work-up is the core of what you do as a student, especially on medical rotations. A good work-up helps you learn and makes you look good. You will find a sample work-up including admission orders in Appendix I, and a case presentation in Appendix II. You will find it helpful to see how our suggestions are used in the sample work-up. When preparing a work-up, many effective scutboys write up everything except the assessment and plans the night of the patient's admission to the hospital, and write the assessment and plans (A&P) the next day when they are a bit more alert. Find out when your complete work-up is expected on the chart. When doing a write-up remember that quality is more important than quantity.

1. *The chief complaint (CC).* Your readers will find your words more useful in understanding the CC than the patient's exact words. You might look upon the CC as an introductory statement about the patient. Some hospitals prefer the patient's exact words.

2. *History of present illness (HPI).* The HPI should be introduced with a sentence or two describing the patient's previous health and his or her most significant past medical history. Accurately note the date of the onset of symptoms. This point needs to be carefully reviewed with the patient.

Patients often relate the onset of an illness to an accident or viral syndrome. You may need to push for clues that the illness may have actually started sooner.

The HPI should be a concise story with a plot that can be followed easily by the reader. Avoid wordy descriptions in lay terms that can be summarized using a short medical phrase (e.g., "paroxysmal nocturnal dyspnea (PND)" instead of "waking up in the middle of the night gasping for breath and feeling terrible ..."). Do not get off the track and discuss unimportant details. You should lead the reader along a direct path that suggests a differential diagnosis (DDx). If available, document results of any previous diagnostic studies such as labs or x-rays.
Pertinent negatives showing that you are already thinking about the DDx should be included at the end of the HPI.

Routinely including this material in your write-up will remind you to be thinking of the DDx as you question the patient. Your *entire* write-up should show that you are considering the DDx throughout your evaluation of the patient.

3. Past medical history (PMH)

    a. *General health:* That is, state of health before the present

    b. *Medical illnesses:* Pneumonia, rheumatic fever, venereal disease, hepatitis, jaundice, tuberculosis, diabetes, hypertension, etc. If a patient says "Yes" to any of these, be sure to inquire further. For example, many people may think that they have had rheumatic fever, but when questioned about symptoms (prolonged illness, joint pains, chest pain, etc.), it becomes clear that they have had some other less severe problem

    c. *Allergies:* Penicillin, sulfa drugs, etc. Be sure to ask and record the exact nature of the adverse reaction. For example, a stomachache as a reaction to penicillin may not be a contraindication to its use, but if the patient says that he or she stopped breathing and was admitted to the hospital, you might think twice

    d. *Hospitalizations and operations* List all hospitalizations in chronological order. Describe procedures, diagnosis, and list physician's name

    e. *Blood transfusions:* Check for adverse reactions

    f. *Serious injuries:* Broken bones, car accidents, etc.

    g. *Drugs* Inquire about the use of alcohol, cigarettes, and any drug abuse

    h. *Present medications:* Include doses and schedule

4. *Family history (FH).* The FH is best shown with a pedigree diagram. Note ages and health problems of immediate relatives. Ask specifically about heart disease, hypertension, stroke, gout, diabetes, thyroid disease, rheumatic disease,

blood disease, kidney disease, asthma, allergies, and sickle cell (if applicable). Also, ask if anyone in the family has any problems similar to the patient's present illness.

5. Social history (SH)
   a. *General:* Birthday, marital status, education, employment, military, toxic exposure, sexual history
   b. *Habits:* Sleeping difficulties, use of coffee or tea
   c. *Home:* Location, others living in home, pets
   d. *Travel:* Especially important if you suspect parasitic and certain other infectious diseases

6. *Review of systems (ROS):* Explain to the patient that you have a long series of questions that you must ask every patient. Each positive answer in this list should have a brief explanation. Those topics covered in the HPI (such as "Skeletal" in a patient admitted with a CC of joint pains) can be dismissed with "see HPI."

Do not take shortcuts with the ROS. List all positives and negatives for now. Even though it is tedious, you must become very familiar with this important part of history taking. Often the most important diagnostic clue may only turn up during a careful ROS.

---

   a. *Skin:* Rashes, itching, change in color, consistency, hair distribution
   b. *Skeletal:* Stiffness, pain, redness, swelling. Record any history of arthritis and length of morning stiffness, if any
   c. *Head*
      (1) *General:* Fainting, headaches, dizziness, head injuries
      (2) *Eyes:* Quality of vision (Are glasses required?), double vision, conjunctivitis, infection, pain, redness, discharge

(3) *Ears:* Quality of hearing, recent decrease in acuity, ringing, infections, pain, blood, discharge, vertigo (distinguished from dizziness as the sensation after getting off a merry-go-round rather than lightheadedness)

(4) *Nose:* Sinus problems, nosebleeds, postnasal drip, sense of smell

(5) *Teeth:* Tooth abcesses, dentures, caries, bleeding gums

(6) *Tongue:* Swelling, pain, sores or ulcers, color, general appearance

(7) *Throat:* Sore throats, difficulty swallowing, history of strep throat

(8) *Neck:* Stiffness, pain, swelling

d. *Endocrine:* Inquire about size of thyroid gland and pain. Ask about the various features of endocrinologic disorders, such as heat intolerance, cold intolerance, polyuria, polydipsia, etc.

e. *Hematologic:* Bleeding problems (as when shaving, brushing teeth), easy bruising, history of anemia or "low blood count"

f. *Lymph nodes:* Ask if the patient has noticed any lumps in the neck, axilla, or groin. If lumps are present, ask if they are painful, red, or draining

g. *Respiratory:* Chest pain (and its relation to breathing), shortness of breath (SOB), cough, sputum production, bloody cough, night sweats (can be seen in TB and a variety of infectious and malignant conditions; in real night sweats, the patient has to change pajamas or bed sheets), exposure to TB. If the patient admits to SOB, pin down exactly what elicits it, such as lying down, walking two blocks, climbing two flights of stairs. Find out what limits the patient. Is it breathing or chest pain? Is the problem severe enough to make the patient stop the activity or can he or she continue exercising?

h. *Cardiac:* Chest pain or *discomfort,* radiation, palpitations, cyanosis, SOB, orthopnea, PND, edema, high blood pressure (HBP). Really try to obtain specific information regarding *when* the patient feels chest discomfort. Exactly what brings it on, where does it hurt, and where does the pain go? Does he or she become nauseated, short of breath, or sweat profusely during the attack? What makes the pain stop? These are all critical questions in deciding if the problem is cardiac, pulmonary, or involves some other system

i. *Gastroenterology:* Appetite, trouble with digestion, heartburn, nausea and vomiting (N&V), hematemesis, diarrhea, constipation, black tarry stools, bloody stools, change in bowel habit, hemorrhoids, ulcers, gallbladder problems, jaundice, dark urine, use of laxatives

j. *GU:* Dysuria, frequency, discharge, hematuria, incontinence, nocturia, difficulty starting stream (particularly for males), flank pain, libido, impotence. *Specifically for female GU:* Age of menarche, regularity of periods, pain, length of period, quantity of flow (in number of tampons or pads per day or cycle), spotting, number of pregnancies, type of contraception, surgery (including abortions), breast pain, lumps, or discharge from nipples

k. *Neuromuscular:* Problems with coordination, weakness, tremor, paralysis, numbness, paresthesias, memory lapses, seizures. Of course, any seizure should be described as accurately as possible

l. *General:* Fevers, chills, recent weight loss or gain. Ask the patient if you have missed any topic

One way to organize the rather lengthy list of symptoms in the ROS is to divide them into positives and negatives for each topic in your write-up. For example:

Respiratory: +   SOB (four blocks, no chest pain, no change in the last 3 years)

— Cough, hemoptysis, chest pain, TB, night sweats

➤ 7. *Physical examination:* There are many ways to organize a physical exam. As you progress you will develop a style that suits you best. We present one way to quickly and efficiently examine your patient. It is a regional rather than a systems approach. This regional approach also keeps manipulation of the patient to a minimum (which becomes important if the patient is in pain or comatose). As you perform your exam, you will think of additional questions to ask the patient.

a. Patient sitting

(1) *Vital signs (VS):* Record the temperature, weight, height (if possible), P (supine and standing), respirations, BP (supine and standing)

Be sure to document whether or not the pulse is regular. Hospitalized patients often develop arrhythmias and knowledge of the original rhythm is important.

---

(2) Hands and arms

(a) *Hands:* Carefully examine the hands and nail beds, being especially watchful for clubbing, splinter hemorrhages, cyanosis, and arthritic changes

---

Get in the habit of flexing and extending the patient's wrists and elbows. Restrictions in these joints may be early evidence of inflammatory arthritis.

(b) *Arms:* Examine skin, muscle tone, and joint range of motion (ROM)

Tophi and rheumatoid nodules are frequently located in the olecranon area.

(c) *Pulses:* Record the intensity of the radial and brachial pulses. While counting the pulse, also check respiratory rate. Don't ask patients to breathe normally because this will make them self-conscious, which may alter the breathing pattern

---

These measurements may be done more easily at the very beginning of the exam or as part of the VS measurements.

(d) *Blood pressure:* Pressures in *both* arms, with patient supine and standing, should be checked

(3) Head
  (a) Examine the skull, scalp, and hair

The scalp is frequently overlooked. If the patient wears a wig, find out why and for how long. Alopecia is a feature of many systemic illnesses.

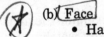

(b) Face
  • Have patient clench teeth, and then palpate temporalis and masseters (CN V)
  • *Pinprick:* Forehead, cheeks, jaw (also light touch) (CN V)
  • Test corneal reflex
  • Have patient raise eyebrows, frown, tightly close eyes, show teeth, smile, puff out cheeks (CN VII)

(4) Eyes

The eye exam is a pivotal part of the neurologic exam, so make a special effort to master it. Additionally, the funduscopic exam is a critical part of the evaluation of diabetes and hypertension and often important in evaluating many other systemic diseases.

(a) *Visual acuity:* Ability to read chart (or finger counting if patient cannot read) in all fields
(b) Position and alignment of eyes, eyelids, and eyebrows
(c) *Conjunctiva:* Look for pallor, hyperemia, discharge
(d) Check extraocular movements (CN III, IV, VI)
(e) *Pupils:* Check for roundness, reaction to light and accommodation, check for Argyll Robertson pupil, diameter. Move your light back and forth between the two eyes to check for Marcus Gunn pupil

---

Pupil size is often noted as a series of three numbers representing the diameter of the pupil in millimeters at rest, exposed to light, and when the opposite pupil is exposed to light.

(f) *Fundoscopic exam:* You may want to dilate the pupils (*after* checking for reflexes and only if pupillary reaction doesn't have to be followed carefully over the next few hours). Look at the optic disk, caliber of arteries and veins, AV crossing, and then check for hemorrhages and exudates. If possible, study the veins carefully for pulsations. This is a better sign for normal CNS pressure than sharp disk margins

---

Becoming comfortable manipulating an ophthalmoscope is not easy. Many novice scutboys practice on friends, spouses, or pets. If you have none of these, simply make a cube of paper (each side 2 to 3 inches), with print on the inside. Make a hole in the wall of the cube opposite the print to simulate the pupil. You can then move the ophthalmoscope to follow and keep in focus the lines of print and become quite adept with the instrument.

---

(5) <u>Ears</u>
- (a) Auricles for tenderness, tophi, signs of infection
- (b) *Hearing (CN VIII):* Use a ticking watch or a tuning fork
- (c) Weber's test and Rinne's test with a tuning fork
- (d) *Otoscope:* Check external canal, color of tympanic membrane, and quality of light reflex

(6) <u>Nose and sinuses</u>
- (a) *Sense of smell (CN I):* If available, use scents like oil of wintergreen
- (b) Examine mucosa and septum with otoscope
- (c) Palpate sinuses for tenderness

(7) <u>Mouth</u>

If the patient has dentures, these must be removed to provide an adequate examination of the mouth.

- (a) Lips
- (b) Buccal mucosa and palate
- (c) Tongue (check for ulcers). Ask patient to stick tongue out (CN XIII). Note color and whether smooth or rough
- (d) Using tongue depressor, ask patient to say "Ah." Watch for symmetric movement of soft palate and uvula. Examine throat and tonsils at this time
- (e) Check gag reflex (usually obvious)

(8) <u>Neck</u>
- (a) Examine cervical lymph nodes

Make it a habit to move your hands down to examine the supraclavicular lymph nodes while examining the cervical lymph nodes.

    (b) Check for tracheal deviation
    (c) Neck flexibility
    (d) Shoulder shrug and head turning against pressure (CN XI)
    (e) Now, with the patient sitting, move behind the patient and examine the thyroid
(9) <u>Back, posterior thorax, and lungs</u>

With easy access to chest x-rays, many clinicians perform only a superficial chest exam. Take the time to learn how to do it right and always correlate physical findings and radiologic findings.

    (a) Inspect and palpate the spine and muscles
    (b) Judge rate and rhythm of breathing
    (c) Observe interspaces for retractions during respirations.
    (d) Palpation
        • Place your palms on the patient's back; ask patient to breathe deeply so you will be able to judge symmetry
        • Check for tactile fremitus (ask patient to say "ninety-nine")
    (e) Percussion
        • Percuss lung fields, noting any areas of dullness or hyperresonance
        • Check level, symmetry, and movement of diaphragm
    (f) *Auscultation:* Listen to quality of breath sounds. Identify wheezes and crackles (carefully noting their location), test vocal fremitus, and E to A egophony
(10) <u>*Breasts:*</u> Should be inspected and palpated with patient sitting and lying down. Be sure to examine for axillary lymph nodes and nipple discharge

b. Patient supine

(1) Heart (have patient lying flat, if possible)

(a) *Inspection:* Observe the precordium for abnormal pulsations or rocking motions. Check for jugular venous distention (JVD) (with patient flat, 30°, 60°, and 90°) and hepatojugular reflux (HJR)

(b) *Palpation:* Note abnormal pulsations, lifts, thrills. Locate point of maximal impulse (PMI) and judge its diameter and intensity. Check for right ventricular lifts and palpable S_3s. Palpate the carotid pulse

(c) *Auscultation (use carotid pulse for timing of systole):*

- Listen at the apex, along the left sternal border (LSB), and upper right sternal border (RSB) with the diaphragm. You should also listen at the axilla. With the bell of the stethoscope listen at the apex, axilla, and lower left sternal border (LLSB). Check for carotid bruits at this time

- When auscultating, listen specifically at each location for S_1, S_2, splitting, gallops, and clicks. Then identify murmurs in systole and diastole

- Listen with the patient sitting up at full expiration (aortic regurgitation (AR) and rubs) and in the left lateral decubitus position (gallops)

Each of these sounds must be sought individually in each location. For example, at each location ask yourself if there is a diastolic murmur. Following this approach will rapidly improve your cardiac exam.

---

(2) Abdomen.
    (a) *Inspection:* Visible peristalsis, pulsations, masses, veins (especially around the umbilicus), protuberance, striae

---

Auscultation of the abdomen is usually performed before palpation because palpation might affect bowel sounds.

    (b) *Auscultation:* Quality of bowel sounds, renal and aortic bruits, rubs
    (c) *Percussion:* Liver (from above and below), stomach bubble, spleen, shifting dullness
    (d) *Palpation:* Liver, spleen. Check for tenderness, guarding, rebound. If possible, palpate kidneys and aorta

---

As part of palpation of the abdomen, rest your hand with mild pressure on the midabdomen to feel the aortic pulsation and to be sure an aneurysm cannot be palpated.

---

(3) *Nodes:* Check inguinal, femoral, axillary, epitrochlear, supraclavicular regions. Listen for femoral bruits and check femoral pulses when checking this region for nodes
(4) Legs
    (a) Pulses
    (b) Edema (pitting)

When checking for pitting edema, be sure to apply pressure for several seconds.

      (c) Examine all joints for fluid, ROM, tenderness

      (d) Look for signs of vascular insufficiency (stasis ulcers, varicose veins, etc.)

  (5) Neurologic

      (a) *Brief mental status:* Orientation, state of consciousness, serial 7s memory, proverbs

      (b) *Cranial nerves:* Already tested!!!

      (c) *Motor:* Tone, bulk, strength of major muscle groups

      (d) *Gait:* Also have patient walk on toes and heels

      (e) Cerebellar

         • Heel-to-toe walking, heel-to-shin, finger-to-nose

         • Rapid alternating movements

      (f) *Sensation:* Pin, light touch, vibration, proprioception, Romberg's test

      (g) Deep tendon reflexes and pathologic reflexes (Babinski's reflex, snout, root, etc.)

Ankle jerks are often difficult to demonstrate. A technique that we have found useful is to have the patient rest the ball of his or her foot on your free hand with the ankle very slightly flexed. Then ask the patient to apply slight pressure on that hand (like pushing the gas pedal driving 2 miles per hour). Using this maneuver, ankle reflexes are usually easily obtained while the patient is applying the slight pressure.

---

  (6) GU

      (a) *Males:* Examine penis, scrotum, testes, and epididymis. Check for varicoceles

      (b) *Females:* Thorough pelvic examination is required on all female patients

  (7) *Rectal:* Sphincter tone, masses, stool, and prostate in males. All patients must have stool tested for occult blood

This format is only a suggestion. You will develop a style on your own. Also, our format is only an outline of the complete physical examination; you will want to expand on various sections depending on the circumstances.

Several points should be made about the proper way to record the physical exam. Although it is generally permissible to dismiss findings as "normal," some normal findings, such as peripheral pulses, should be carefully documented.

Beginning students are expected to completely describe even normal findings to ensure that a careful exam and proper descriptions are being learned.

- Begin with a brief general description of the patient, including race, sex, general appearance, state of discomfort or distress, abnormal breathing or altered mental status. Then list the VS. In general, the description of the exam follows the same order in which you performed it
- *Skin:* Should have been noted throughout the exam. Carefully describe lesions
- Skeletal
- HEENT
- *Lymph nodes:* In any case of infection or possible neoplasm, the presence or absence of adenopathy must be carefully documented
- Neck
- Breasts
- Lungs
- Cardiovascular
- Peripheral pulses
- *Abdomen:* Record liver span (in centimeters) and the presence or absence of palpable spleen

- *Neurologic:* Stick diagrams are useful for DTRs and motor exam. Try to avoid statements such as "neurologic exam physiologic" or "cranial nerves II through XII intact." The latter is seen quite frequently and is a time-saver, but should be avoided, especially in a patient with a neurologic problem who needs a carefully documented exam
- GU and rectal

8. *Labs:* The five lab studies listed below are the basic ones that go in most work-ups. Others may be added when appropriate (e.g., blood gases). All lab studies should be charted before morning rounds. You may wish to include a description of the peripheral blood smear here.

These labs may be too expensive to obtain routinely in this era of cost containment. But scutboy time is cheap. Labs performed by you, e.g., urinalysis, are virtually free.

---

a. *Urinalysis:* Gross appearance, specific gravity (sg), dipstick (pH, protein, glucose, ketose, bilirubin, blood), sulfasalic acid (SSA), sediment (RBC, WBC, bacteria, casts). The dipstick for protein tests only for albumin, but SSA tests for any protein, (e.g., Bence Jones protein) and should therefore be included in a routine urinalysis. Simply squirt some SSA solution into 1 to 2 cc of urine; a white precipitate forms if the test is positive.

For a proper microscopic exam, fresh (less than 1 hour old) clean-catch urine should be used. Spin the urine in a centrifuge for 1 to 2 minutes, pour of the urine, resuspend the sediment by banging the test tube against some convenient surface. Place a drop of the resuspended sediment on a slide and add a coverslip. Casts are best looked for at low power, around the edges of the coverslip. Use the high-dry power (40 × lens) to look at cells. Bacteria are often crudely quantitated at the 1+ to 4+ and cells as the number seen per high-power field.

b. *SMA-6:* This consists of the serum electrolytes (Na, K, Cl, HCO$_3$) and the BUN and creatinine (or glucose at some hospitals). It is often written thus:

Na	Cl	BUN
K	HCO$_3$	Creatinine

Different hospitals use different terminology for the same panel of labs. The SMA-6 is also known as M-6, chem panel, chem 6, and electrolyte panel.

c. *Hematology:* Hct; WBC; RBC; red cell indices; differential WBC count; platelet count (not always necessary if "adequate" on peripheral smear); protime (PT) and (PTT) if indicated

d. *Chest x-ray:* A brief description (be sure to look at the CXR yourself)

e. *ECG:* Rate, rhythm, axis, intervals, (PR, QRS, QT), hypertrophy, signs of infarct or ischemia, followed by your interpretation of the ECG

9. *Assessment (or impressions):* This section may be combine with "Plans" as described in the next section. Along with the HPI, the A&P are the areas in which the student should strive to develop a clear, concise style. First, you should list *all* of the patient's problems, in order of importance. Under each problem there should be a *discussion* of the DDx (i.e., any of the conditions that might be causing the problem). Inactive problems do not need a discussion. (Refer to the example in Appendix I for further discussion.)

10. *Plans:* Your plans regarding each problem should be listed. Plans are of two types, diagnostic and therapeutic, and these may be listed separately. Your plans do not need to be those actually carried out; simply try to think of what you would do if the patient were completely yours.

A word about efficiency: Obviously, doing all of this will take quite a bit of time unless you work very efficiently. Usually the intern will see the patient before you do; however, at some schools, the student sees the patient first. A big time-saver is the practice of writing the PMH, FH, SH, and ROS *as* you talk to the patient. That leaves you with only the physical exam, HPI, and labs to write after you finish seeing the patient (as well as the A&P, of course).

C. PROGRESS NOTES

You should write daily progress notes on all of your patients. Progress notes should not be looked upon as a chore; rather, sitting down at the end of the day with your charts affords you an opportunity to gather your thoughts about each patient.

Since your peers and the house staff will judge how well you are following your patients by your progress notes, these notes must convey a clear idea of what is going on with the patient. Notes should be concise and to the point; do not be afraid to write a brief note. Often several sentences are enough.

The object of a progress note is to convey what has happened to the patient since the previous note and to record your current thinking.

Although many scutboys choose not to use strict SOAP (subjective, objective, assessment, plans) format, several lessons can be learned from the problem-oriented approach:

1. Organize your notes around the patient's problems. Label each part of the note according to the problem being covered and fully discuss that problem before moving on to the next. This approach does wonders for achieving organization.

2. The first part of the discussion of each problem will be an update of what is happening with the patient, including new information from the history, changes in physical exam (or documentation of lack of change), results of lab or other diagnostic studies, new therapy and any response to therapy (be sure to review the orders to make sure you are not forgetting to mention any changes in therapy).

3. Next, discuss your impressions at this point in the patient's progress. Close the note by mentioning what you have planned for treatment, or any planned diagnostic studies. Any abnormal lab or exam findings should be discussed.

After completing the note, look back over it and ask yourself two questions: (1) Will the reader be able to understand what has happened to the patient since the previous note? and (2) Will the reader be able to understand your interpretation of what these developments mean?

The way physicians interpret developments is often more important than the developments themselves. Remember that consultants depend on your progress notes to understand the course of your patients. If you want good consults, write good progress notes.

D. SPECIAL TYPES OF PROGRESS NOTES

1. *Procedure note:* A procedure note is written whenever an invasive procedure (e.g., lumbar puncture (LP), central venous line placement) is performed. The note should include:
   a. Name of the procedure
   b. Date and time procedure was performed
   c. Indication for procedure
   d. How the procedure was carried out (including such information as the patient's position, size of needles used) and by whom
   e. Any apparent complications and how the procedure was tolerated by the patient

f. Results and any observations made during the procedure. A description of any fluid obtained should be included

Procedure notes are usually written by the person performing the procedure.

Sometimes a procedure is performed as part of a consult and the procedure note is written on a separate consult sheet outside of the regular progress notes or might even be dictated. In that case a quick notation such as "Procedure—see consult sheet" should be made in the progress notes. That way if the patient's condition should change suddenly, someone quickly looking at the chart will be aware of all recent procedures.

---

2. *Consult note:* Most hospitals have special forms on which consults are written. Often consultants also write notes in the regular progress note section. On basic rotations, you will not be writing consult notes. However, when your turn comes to write these notes keep these points in mind:

a. *Answer the question being asked:* When requesting a consult try to ask the consultant as specific a question as possible. For example, when ordering a cardiology consult you might ask about which antiarrhythmic drug is best for a patient rather than simply "evaluate patient." As a consultant try to figure out exactly what the primary physician wants to know. Obviously the best solution is for the primary physician and the consultant to talk *before* the consult—another reason to call in your own consults.

b. *Be brief and specific:* Somewhere in the consult note there should be a specific list of recommendations. Students tend to write very detailed consult notes which no one wants to wade through to find the exact recommendations.

c. *Be prompt:* Even if you need a day or two to give a final opinion (usually because the attending consultant may only round on certain days), try to give a brief list of recommendations quickly. In particular, recommend important diagnostic tests promptly.

3. *Off-service note:* When a physician changes services, monthly for most interns, a note should be written for the benefit of the incoming physician. This note should include a brief discussion of the patient's initial presentation, the hospital course, results of important studies, a current pertinent physical exam, current medications, and a list of the active problems and plans. Although house staff usually write the notes, you might be expected to as well.

4. *Transfer note:* When a patient is transferred from one service to another, e.g., from medicine to surgery or from ward to ICU, a transfer note is written which follows the same format as an off-service note. As a student it is likely you will be expected to write these notes for your patients if they are transferred to another service.

5. *On-service note or transfer acceptance note:* These are notes written by the physician coming "on service" or on the receiving end of a transfer. The purpose of the note is to convey an understanding of the patient's problems and should include a physical exam.

6. *Operative notes:* Pre-op, brief-op, and post-op notes are discussed in "Surgery Rotation," pp. 46–51.

7. *Discharge summary:* This is a brief summary of the hospital course, to be written at the time of discharge. Usually the intern or resident will have to dictate the note, but it is a good idea for you to write one also. A brief handwritten discharge summary is an incredible help to the house officer dictating and will put you in his or her good graces forever.

The format is as follows:

   a. One or two sentences explaining why the patient was admitted
   b. *Hospital course:* Be *brief* and specific while recounting the patient's work-up. Include pertinent laboratory data
   c. *Operations:* List the date and type of procedure(s) (including LPs, thoracenteses, etc.)
   d. Discharge medicines (include dosages)
   e. *Discharge diagnoses:* This is simply a list of the patient's problems (e.g., #1 myocardial infarction, #2 anemia, etc.)
   f. *Disposition:* State where the patient is going (e.g., home, nursing home, etc.)
   g. Patient's condition upon discharge
   h. *Follow up:* State the name of the physician who will follow the patient

Aim for a note that is only one or two pages long. If it's too long no one will read it. If it's too short, it's useless.

Often a brief physical exam should be included in the summary documenting physical findings at discharge. For example, a patient who has undergone a neurologic operation should have a neurologic exam documented at the time of discharge. This is of great importance if the patient should become ill or develop a complication.

E. OUTPATIENT NOTES

Although most medical students' rotations are oriented around inpatient services, some include a clinic experience. Although new (to the clinic) patient notes are very similar to your standard admission write-up, return visit notes are far more concise. Unfortunately, vital information is often left out, leaving many clinic notes virtually useless. Clinic notes for returning patients should include:

1. *Problem list:* In some clinics, an "official" problem list is kept in the chart. If so, be sure that it is current. If not, list the patient's problems prominently.

Not only will an accurate and current list of problems help the next person who sees the patient, it will prevent you from overlooking important information.

---

2. *Medications:* Carefully review the medication list with the patient, then carefully explain doses. You will be amazed how often it is impossible to figure out what a patient is supposed to be taking from reviewing a chart.

Whenever you start a new medication, clearly explain if any of the patient's previous medications should be stopped. Patients often assume that a new medicine is replacing an old one.

It is a good idea to have your patients bring all of their medicine with them for clinic visits so that you can review them carefully.

---

3. Note VS and the general appearance of the patient

4. Update each problem with both subjective (historical) and objective (exam, labs) information.

You will not be performing a complete physical exam on each patient so clearly document exactly what you do examine. Try to avoid generalizations such as "neurologic exam normal" because that does not provide a clear baseline for subsequent examinations.

---

5. Briefly discuss your assessment of the current status of each problem and list your plans. Carefully note any medication changes.

6. State when the patient is to return to the clinic. Whenever studies are planned, be sure that you will be promptly notified of the results. That may mean calling the lab yourself. Amazingly, many clinics do not have a mechanism for notifying physicians of lab results.

F. ORDERS

Physicians' orders are the means by which patient care is directed. All orders that you write will need to be countersigned by the patient's intern. You should strive to write all orders on your patients.

In general, orders are very easy to write, although there are a couple of instances in which a special format is used.

Admission orders are written as soon as possible after a new patient reaches the floor. There is nothing sacred about the sequence used here, but the orders should include:

1. *Admit to:* Name of floor; name of attending

2. *Diagnosis:* e.g., Diabetes

3. *Condition:* e.g., stable; critical

4. *Allergies:* e.g., penicillin

5. *VS:* You should state how frequently VS are to be taken (e.g., q shift); any special instructions (e.g., rectal temps). It is wise to get VS q4h for the first 24 hours to be sure the patient is stable

6. *Activity:* e.g., ad lib; bedrest

7. *Diet:* e.g., 1500 calorie ADA

8. *IV orders:* IV bottles should be numbered and instructions as to rate and times given. For example:

#1   ILD5 0.2 NS + 20 mEq KCl over 12 hr, 3 A.M. → 3 P.M.
#2   ILD5 0.2 NS + 20 mEq KCl over 12 hr, 3 P.M. → 3 A.M.
You may also write for 24 hours of IV fluids at one time.

You may request that the IV team start an IV (if such a service is available in your hospital); be sure to specify what type of IV you want (e.g., IV team to start IV with #18 angiocath in either arm). Orders for IV fluids may also be written by specifying rate and duration of the infusion (e.g., D5½ NS + 20 mEq KCl/L at 100 cc/h x 24 h.)

9. *Medications:* Specify name, dosage, route, frequency (e.g., digoxin 0.25 mg p.o. q.d.)

10. *Labs:* (e.g., request A.M. bloods)

11. *Special nursing:* e.g., physical therapy; restraints)

12. *"Scare orders":* These specify parameters for the nurses and indicate when the intern should be notified (e.g., temperature >38C, BP >170/110, BP <90/50, P >120 or <50)

Discharge orders should include these items:

- Discharge in A.M. (or today)
- Diagnosis
- *Disposition:* e.g., home
- *Medicines:* Listed with dosages
- Follow-up

All orders should be dated and should include the time when written. See Appendix III, "Sample Admission Orders."

G. PRESENTING CASES

The ability to present cases well is heavily stressed by the faculty and house staff. There is nothing difficult about presenting a case as long as a few principles are remembered:

1. The key to a good case is brevity. Organization is important; in order for a presentation to be brief it must be well organized. Only mention absolutely pertinent facts.

2. Aim for a 2- to 4-minute presentation (that is not much time).

3. If presenting to an attending, have all pertinent x-rays and ECGs present (e.g., if you are presenting a patient with pneumonia have the chest x-ray with you).

4. Begin the presentation with an introductory statement similar to the CC in your write-up (refer to Appendix I). However, a presentation is not an oral rendition of your write-up; it is a carefully edited version.

5. Next, give a sentence or two about the patient's PMH. (You may wait until after discussing the HPI, but a brief summary of the PMH at the outset will help familiarize your listeners with your patient).

6. Now give a *concise* HPI, keeping in mind the rules given for the write-up. This is the most important part of the presentation and will usually take about one third to one half of your time. Organization is critical.

7. Next say, "The past medical history, family history, social history, and review of systems were otherwise noncontributory."

8. One essential point should be made now: If you open an issue, close it! For example, if you say, "The patient was treated for hyperthyroidism by thyroidectomy 10 years ago," your next sentence should be, "and he has had no symptoms of thyroid disease since that time." Do not leave your listeners wondering about thyroid when you move on to the next topic. This rule may seem obvious, but you will be amazed at how often it is broken.

9. Your description of the physical exam should begin with a general description of the patient.

At some hospitals, presentations are made at the bedside so that the patient is in view. Under that circumstance, do not say things that are obvious, such as the patient's race and sex. Instead start the presentation with the patient's age and occupation. Avoid statements like "The patient appeared much as you see him now."

10. Next, give the vital signs (most house officers and attendings prefer to hear what the vital signs were—not just "VS were WNL").

11. In describing the physical exam itself, mention only those findings that are directly relevant to the HPI. No one wants to hear a string of normal findings unless they are absolutely pertinent.

12. You may conclude the physical exam description by stating, "The remainder of the physical exam was unremarkable." This reminds your grateful listeners that you mentioned only the most relevant findings.

13. Laboratory values should be dismissed as normal whenever possible. No one wants to hear about electrolytes if they are normal unless they have a direct bearing on the case.

14. After the lab results are given, you should make a statement summarizing the patient so that your listeners will know that you are finished.

15. At this point you may wish to describe any action taken in the immediate management of the patient or your A&P. Usually one of your listeners will want to hear this additional information and will ask for it.

16. Do not think that your presentation is incomplete if you are questioned. A good presentation will stir enough interest in your listeners for them to ask questions.

17. You will probably never be criticized for making a presentation too brief. The most common error students make in presenting cases is making the presentation too long.

H. WRITING PRESCRIPTIONS

Whether working in an outpatient setting or discharging inpatients, you will be expected to write medication prescriptions. This task requires great care because medication errors commonly result from incorrect, incomplete, or illegible prescriptions. Print if you must to be legible. Always proofread the prescription before giving it to the patient. A prescription consists of the following information:

1. *Patient's name and date:* Leaving off either of these will make a prescription invalid. Pharmacists will not fill a prescription for a Schedule II drug, such as a narcotic, over 10 days old.

2. *Superscription:* The symbol R is usually printed on prescription forms and is an abbreviation for the Latin *recipe* (take thou). This symbol precedes the name of the prescribed medication.

3. *Name of drug:* In some states, use of a proprietary or brand name obligates the pharmacist to dispense the exact brand that you prescribe. In other states, notation by the physician such as "dispense as written" or "substitution permitted" determines whether the brand name is dispensed. Find out what your state regulations are.

4. *Dosage:* Some medications are manufactured in only one dose whereas others are manufactured in several doses or preparations. Always specify which dose you are prescribing.

5. *Amount of the medication to be dispensed:* Write this as disp. or "#" and give the amount, e.g., number of tablets to be dispensed.

6. *Instructions:* The instructions to the patient for how to take the medication follow the abbreviation *sig.* (for *signa* or label). Most pharmacists recommend that these instructions be written in English, but most physicians use Latin abbreviations. In either case, the pharmacist will translate your instructions into English for the label. Often, stating the purpose of the medication after the specific instructions is helpful in familiarizing the patient with the medicine.

7. *Refill information:* Specify the number of times the prescription can be refilled.

8. *Signature:* As a student, you will need to have all the prescriptions you write signed by a licensed physician. His drug enforcement adminstration (DEA) number will usually be added (required for Schedule II drugs).

9. Sample prescription

Johnny Rotten, M.D.
DEA No. AR1234567

Name *Joey Ramone* _____ Age _____

Address _____ Date 5·22·87

R *Naprosyn 500mg tabs #60*
   sig: ℞ tab b.i.d. for arthritis

Refill *one* times

J Rotten, M.D.

_____   _____
Substitution permitted   Dispense as written

I. "PERIPHERAL BRAINS" FOR THE STUDENT

You will find that being chronically overworked and exhausted does not help your memory. Therefore, you will need to carry a few "crutches" with you to help keep things straight.

The first item is a *scutpad.* (Some students prefer a clipboard; others use cards.) The scutpad is used to keep track of everything that you need to do for each patient. Write down scut as soon as someone tells you to do something or you think of something to do, so that you don't forget anything.

Patient index cards are also invaluable. You need to carry your patients' history numbers with you, and this is one way to do it. On the index card you may also write a summary of each patient's work-up to read over before presenting a case.

Many people keep a *pocket-sized notebook* (which they carry next to a copy of *The Effective Scutboy)* that contains clinical pearls such as dosages of commonly used medicines, phone numbers, etc. Such a notebook will work wonders for a failing memory.

Don't be afraid to ask the house officers for help. They are generally delighted to help students.

J. RECOMMENDED READING

This section might be more appropriately titled "Recommended Buying." Deciding which textbooks to buy is increasingly difficult because there are so many books available and they are increasingly expensive (medical textbooks are probably second only to medical school tuition in the inflation sweepstakes—sure we can laugh, we already graduated). Ten years ago a student could buy the major textbook for each specialty. Today that is not necessarily the best approach. A number of books have appeared that are far more succinct and practical than the major textbooks. A reasonable strategy now is to buy a good paperback to read for each rotation and use major textbooks (borrowed or from the library) as a reference. As for specific recommendations:

- *The Effective Scutboy,* 3/E, by Harrell and Firestein. A classic in its own time and a must for serious students. This book should be bought, not borrowed.
- *The Principles and Practice of Medicine,* 22/E, by Harvey, et al. Originally written by Sir William Osler, this book had a major impact on the practice of medicine and medical education. It remains the best textbook of internal medicine for students. This book is intended to be a text—not a reference. While other books can be used to look up details of specific diseases, this book can (and should) be read cover to cover. We liked it even before its publisher began publishing the *Scutboy.*
- *Major internal medicine textbook.* Although collecting fat textbooks is not the goal here, you do need a comprehensive internal medicine text as a reference book. The major selections are Cecil, Stein, and Harrisons. They are authored by many recognized experts and in our opinion are probably equivalent. Buy the one that is most current.
- *Rapid Interpretation of ECG* by Dubin. The fastest way to develop competence interpreting ECGs. After a few hours with this book you too can read ECGs.
- *Practical Electrocardiography* by Marriott. After Dubin, read this. It also makes a useful reference for virtually all ECGs you will encounter.
- *New England Journal of Medicine.* If you give in to the urge to subscribe to a journal, this is a good choice. It arrives weekly, so it forms an impressive looking stack in no time. The CPCs are quite good, the original articles important, and the editorials worth reading. However, most of the major articles will appear in your local newspaper (in a condensed and easy-to-read form). Subscribing to the newspaper will also keep you up-to-date with sports, comics, etc. You decide which you would rather have.

- *Neurology for the House Officer* by Weiner and Levitt. This is perhaps the most popular book of the "For the House Officer" series of books. It is very practical and actually has as much useful information as most of the large neurology texts.
- *Manual of Medical Therapeutics* by the Washington University Department of Medicine. The "Washington Manual" has become the universal "pocket resident" since its introduction in 1950. New editions appear about every 3 years. This book provides essential information for managing most medical problems and often has useful diagnostic information as well. If you knew everything in this book, you would be a stellar physician. This book has spawned the entire "Little, Brown Spiral Manual" series, most of which are very good and now numbers over 50 titles.
- *Problem-Oriented Medical Diagnosis* by Friedman. Another of the Little, Brown series, this book nicely complements the "Washington Manual" by providing diagnostic information, in particular excellent differential diagnoses, for a wide range of medical problems. The suggested work-ups are at times overly extensive, but they do provide a good framework to help you organize your own plans for a given patient.
- *Guide to Antimicrobial Therapy* by Sanford. A real bargain! For about $5.00 you get a pocket-sized book with over 100 pages of essential information about infectious diseases and the ever-changing world of antibiotics. Most of the information is presented in easy to follow tables and charts. If not available at your bookstore, it can be ordered from the author, Jay P. Sanford, M.D., P.O. Box 34456, West Bethesda, Maryland, 20817-0456. New edition available every year.
- *Primer on the Rheumatic Diseases* by the Arthritis Foundation. Speaking of bargains, this book is free! Written by a panel of experts, here is a 200+ page rheumatology

textbook that can be obtained merely by requesting (check with your rheumatology department). If unavailable locally, write to the Arthritis Foundation, 1314 Spring Street N.W., Atlanta, Georgia 30309.

- *The Effective Clinician* by Tumulty. Here is an opportunity to learn how a master clinician (and author of our introduction) approaches patients. This book should be read several times during your career—you will take away something new every time. If it's not in your bookstore, check the library.
- *Guide to Physical Examination and History Taking* by Bates. This book keeps getting better and better. It is probably the best book available to help you learn how to perform the physical exam.
- *Bedside Diagnostic Examination* by DeGowin. More comprehensive than Bates and more portable, this book is an excellent reference, but probably not as useful an introductory text. However, in a year or two you will use it more than Bates.
- *Fundamentals of Radiology* by Squire. This book has been around for ages and will not teach you the latest radiology techniques. However, spending several evenings with this book is a good way to develop some real confidence reading chest x-rays and improve your basic ability with other standard x-rays.
- *Diagnosis of Stupor and Coma* by Plum and Posner. Now available in a soft-cover edition, this book is very useful in understanding the central nervous system and seeing what all of that neuroanatomy you memorized is about.
- *House of God* by Shem. If you want your friends and relatives to understand the dark side of medical training, this book is a must. The plot may not be realistic, but it portrays the frustration of modern medical training. Read it now; it will not be as much fun once you are an intern.

Whenever we visit a medical bookstore we are amazed at the explosion of new paperback medical books (we may be in part to blame—some of them are imitations of *The Effective Scutboy*). Several good series of books, in addition to the Little, Brown and "For the House Officer" series, are available. You are probably familiar with the Lange Series and their excellent basic science books. They also have a group of "Handbooks" for the major clinical specialties that are quite good. Saunders produces a spiral-bound Blue Book series. Many small books are too brief, often little more than lists. You need books with a bit more flesh. Since there are now several nice small texts for any rotation you should have no trouble finding one you like. If you find anything really special, please write to us in care of our publisher and we will pass on your recommendations in the next edition.

K. COMMONLY ENCOUNTERED MANAGEMENT PROBLEMS

Constipation, insomnia, and pain are problems for almost all inpatients and many outpatients. This section is designed to give you an overview of the medications commonly used for them. Many scutboys routinely write p.r.n. orders for all three of these problems as part of their admission orders for all patients. Obviously, becoming comfortable in treating these conditions is essential. Remember that these are only suggestions, and that you should never prescribe a drug without consulting a physician. You should be familiar with all medications that you prescribe, including their side effects. The dosages suggested here are standard, but all dosages should be checked before you prescribe a medicine. A house officer will *always* need to approve any medications you wish to prescribe.

1. *Constipation:* You will be shocked at patients' preoccupation with their bowels. When patients complain of constipa-

tion, you have a large armamentarium available for treating the condition. In the back of your mind you should always consider the probable *cause* of a patient's constipation, as the cause can affect the drug selection.

The suggested schema is in approximately increasing strength as you move down the list.

a. *Remove known causes of constipation:* This includes opiates and aluminum-containing antacids. Remember that hypercalcemia, spinal compression, and hypothyroidism can cause severe constipation and do not forget that colon cancer can be a cause. The most common cause of constipation in hospitalized patients is probably a combination of inactivity, strange food, and medication

b. *High-fiber diet:* Unfortunately difficult to find in hospitals

c. *Metamucil:* This is a bulk-forming agent that works for mild constipation. Dose: 1 tablespoon in water q.d. or b.i.d.

d. *Colace (or DOSS):* This stool softener is better as a preventive measure and rarely works in a patient already constipated. Dose: 100 to 200 mg p.o. q.d. or b.i.d.

e. *Milk of Magnesia (MOM), magnesium citrate, magnesium antacids* (e.g., *Mylanta, Maalox):* These are excellent cathartics and are often the first-line drugs. *Never give these to patients with renal failure* (beware of hypermagnesemia). We suggest starting with 30 cc of MOM once or twice a day. Mag citrate looks like 7-Up and works like a charm. Mag citrate is a strong laxative and should generally not be your first choice for treatment.

f. *Dulcolax:* The "Duke" is another favorite of ours. This is a gut stimulant that can be given orally or as a rectal suppository. *Don't give this if you suspect mechanical obstruction.* Suppositories usually give results within an hour, while the oral form may take a little longer. The usual suppository dose is q.d. p.r.n. Up to three pills can be taken orally at one time. Occasionally you may be pushed to give the "Double Duke," i.e., Dulcolax from above and below!

g. Enemas

(1) *Fleet:* This is a small enema that can evacuate the rectum (comes commercially prepared). It contains lots of phosphate, so beware in renal failure!

(2) *Soapsuds and tap water:* Large volumes of fluid can be used, and the patient's entire colon can be cleared. Usually the order for these is simply: "Tap water enema until clear." Your patient will either love you or hate you for ordering this.

h. *Disimpaction:* This is the last resort. You need lubricant, gloves, and a strong stomach. *Note:* If the patient appears to be impacted on initial exam, this is the treatment of choice. Remember to double glove.

i. *Rosenfield's maneuver:* Eat a mouse, sit on a piece of cheese. Never fails.

j. Our usual approach is (a) Colace or Metamucil to prevent constipation; (b) MOM; (c) Mag citrate, Dulcolax or enema.

2. *Insomnia:* Although drug dependence is not as much a worry in the hospital as it is with outpatients, care should be taken when prescribing benzodiazepines. Beware that drug interactions producing undesirable levels of sedation are common (e.g., antidepressants and muscle relaxants).

a. Benzodiazepines

(1) *Dalmane:* The most commonly used, because of a large advertising budget. However, it has long-acting metabolites; it can be a respiratory depressant. Dose: 30 mg p.o. q.h.s. (15 mg for the elderly)

(2) *Valium:* As effective as Dalmane, but has the same problem with metabolites. Dose: 5 or 10 mg p.o. q.h.s.

    (3) *Serax* (oxazepam): Has the advantage of having no active metabolites, but may take longer for maximum effect. Dose: 15 to 30 mg p.o. q.h.s.

    (4) *Halcion:* 0.125 to 0.25 mg p.o. q.h.s. Short half-life, but effective

b. *Barbiturates:* Seconal is the one most frequently prescribed. Remember that this will stimulate microsomal enzymes and affect the metabolism of other drugs. *These are addicting.* The dangers of these drugs usually outweigh their usefulness for insomnia and their use should generally be discouraged

c. *Antihistamines:* Anyone who has ever taken a hay fever pill can attest to its sedating action. These are especially useful for outpatients since they are unlikely to cause dependence

    (1) *Benadryl:* 25 or 50 mg; may be given p.o., IM, or IV

    (2) *Hydroxyzine:* 25 or 50 mg

d. *Neuroleptics:* These need to be given with care, especially in the elderly, or the patient may sleep for a couple of days. Prolonged use of phenothiazines can cause tardive dyskinesia, a peculiar syndrome with involuntary facial and tongue movements

    (1) *Haldol:* The drug of choice for elderly patients who "Sun Down" (become agitated and confused at night). Start with 1 or 2 mg IM or p.o. q8h and gradually increase the dose

    (2) *Thorazine:* Use 10 to 25 mg IM or p.o. *Watch for orthostatic hypotension.* You probably shouldn't use this in the geriatric population

e. *Chloral hydrate:* This old standby is better known as a "Mickey Finn" and is very effective. Tolerance can occur. Dose: 500 mg to 1000 mg p.o. q.h.s. Chloral hydrate has a very rapid onset and is cheap. Those who have seen *The Maltese Falcon* know how well it worked on Bogart

Often it helps to ask what the patient usually takes for sleep. Finally, although we do not encourage use of "sleeping pills," people have difficulty sleeping in the strange environment of the hospital; you should not hesitate to help them in the short run. We usually use chloral hydrate or a short-acting benzodiazepine like Halcion.

3. *Pain control:* Pain control is a complex issue, and a variety of modalities are available to the physician. Clear differentiation must be made between chronic and acute pain because these are treated differently. Patients with acute pain, as in postsurgical pain, should be treated with adequate amounts of narcotics. Chronic pain is often managed with nonopiates. One exception to this rule is pain secondary to terminal cancer. Adequate analgesia is essential to patient care in this case. Finally, you often have to explain to patients that drugs do not eliminate pain; they only make the pain bearable. Of course, the cause of pain should be determined before the pain is masked by analgesics. In some circumstances (e.g., acute abdomen) analgesics may be contraindicated.

   a. *Acetaminophen (Tylenol):* This is the first-line drug for mild pain. It has none of the adverse effects of aspirin (gastric irritation, antiplatelet activity) but similar analgesia. Large doses are *hepatotoxic.* Remember that fevers will be suppressed. Dose: 650 mg p.o. or p.r.n. q4h

   b. *Aspirin:* Not used very often now that Tylenol is available. However, if you desire an anti-inflammatory effect, this is the cheapest drug around. Dose: 650 mg p.o. q4h

---

The anti-inflammatory dose of aspirin is often 16 to 20 tablets per day, far higher than an analgesic dose.

---

   c. *Nonsteroidal anti-inflammatory drugs (NSAID):* This class of drugs can be useful for managing mild to moderate pain. The drugs have the advantage of not being addictive. A variety, such as Naprosyn, Motrin, and Indocin, are available. There are many potential side effects, including ulcers, headaches, and renal failure. They should not be prescribed for people who are allergic to aspirin, as there is some cross-reaction

---

NSAIDs should be used with great caution in the elderly and patients with abnormal renal function. Most of these drugs have similar side effects (mostly GI), but Indocin, in particular, often causes CNS disturbances or headaches.

---

   d. Opiates: *Remember that these suppress respiration!*
      (1) *Codeine:* This is the weakest opiate. Nausea is a common side effect
      (2) *Tylenol and codeine:* An effective combination (called Tylenol No. 2, No. 3 or No. 4 depending on the amount of codeine)
      (3) *Darvon (and Darvon and Tylenol):* Useful for mild analgesia if the patient becomes nauseated by codeine
      (4) *Vicodin—*hydrocodone and acetaminophen: Has lesser frequency of nausea than codeine but popular with drug dependent patients
      (5) *Demerol, Dilaudid, Percodan:* Potent narcotics with abuse potential
      (6) *Methadone:* Available for IV or p.o. administration. One important aspect of methadone is that its analgesic half-life is only 4 to 6 hours (although it can suppress withdrawal symptoms for 24 to 36 hours). For maximum pain control, it must be given on a regular q4-6h schedule
      (7) *Morphine:* Can be given IM, subcutaneously, or IV. This potent analgesic is pretty much the gold standard. The dose varies depending on the route

of administration. Terminal cancer patients may benefit from continuous morphine IV infusion

All opiates can be rapidly reversed with an intravenous injection of Narcan. Remember that narcotics cause constipation. Colace may be useful—an ounce of prevention is worth a pound of cure.

L. SURGERY ROTATION

Mark W. Woodruff

The surgery rotation, besides being an exposure to the field of surgery and its subspecialties, will offer you an opportunity to improve your speed in every aspect of medical student responsibility. Patient evaluations, write-ups, and presentations all need to be done in shorter order, simply because there is less time for all of this work given the demands of observing (and it is hoped, helping) in the OR.

A note on the OR experience: Different students feel this rotation is of more or less importance, as do different programs. The one universal guide is that you should spend enough time there to become comfortable with sterile technique because it is relevant to all specialties of medicine.

The primary way to become faster, besides practice, is to be more focused and brief. If the patient is there for a breast biopsy, don't get lost in consideration of her osteoarthritis. In fact at most schools, any medical problem not directly relevant to the patient's surgical problem should be dealt with only briefly in the H&P, and not at all in the rounds presentation.

The exceptions to this rule of thumb are medical problems significant to anesthesia risk, such as cardiac or pulmonary disease, and those that may complicate postoperative care, such as hypertension, poor nutritional status or a history of thrombophlebitis. These should get slightly more attention, including a mention in the presentation.

1. *Admission history and physical examination:* You will use essentially the same format as for any other H&P, except

as already stated, both the Hx and PE should be more directed. Give slightly more prominence to past surgical history than you would otherwise. Remember, surgeons will be more impressed with two completed work-ups than a seven-point assessment with detailed plan of treatment.

If available from the old record, it's useful to include in your history any surgical procedure the patient may have had in the past.

---

2. *Admission orders:* Again, a standard format may be used. If a patient is being admitted for surgery the next day, you must order all preparations at the time of admission, in addition to the routine orders:
   a. *Preoperative labs:* Electrolytes, BUN, creatinine, CBC, PT/PTT, ECG (for patients over 40), CXR (within the last month for patients over 40), unrinalysis; possibly type and cross (T&C) or hold clot in blood bank; consider ABG or PFT for patients with long smoking history or COPD

It may be helpful to specify labs as preoperative on your admission orders because many hospitals have special rapid reporting mechanisms for these results (especially ECG and CXR).

---

   b. N.P.O. after midnight
   c. Void on call to OR
   d. Prep and shave surgical field (this is done in the OR in some institutions to reduce risk of folliculitis which would require cancelling the surgery; this is especially true for surgeries involving prostheses—vascular or orthopedic)
   e. *Other possible preparation for OR:* Antiseptic shower, bowel clean-out, chest PT and pulmonary toilet for patients with COPD, transfusion if patient is anemic,

antibiotic phrophylaxis if indicated, correction of electrolyte abnormalities, etc.

   f. *Preoperative medications, such as a sedative:* These are often ordered by the anesthesiologist, who also sees the patient before the surgery

---

If it's not contraindicated, most patients will appreciate it if you order a bedtime hypnotic ("sleeper") as a p.r.n. medication. Many people have trouble sleeping the night before surgery. Mention that this help is available so the patient will know to ask for it if needed.

---

  3. *Preoperative check:* This is a note written in the chart, usually on the night before surgery. When you are on call, it may be your responsibility to write these. The note itself is not as important as what it signifies: That you have personally made sure everything is in order for your patient to go to the OR the next morning. A sample note includes the following information:

   a. *Preoperative diagnosis:* Cholelithiasis
   b. *Procedure:* Cholecystectomy with intraoperative cholangiogram
   c. *Consent:* Signed
   d. *ECG:* WNL
   e. *CXR:* Clear

You should get some sort of official clearance for the ECG and CXR, or at least check with your resident. You should also call the blood bank to make sure they have the blood.

---

   f. *Labs:* $\dfrac{139 \mid 103 \mid 12}{4.1 \mid 28 \mid 0.8} \diagdown 97 \qquad 205 \equiv \diagup \diagdown \dfrac{13.0}{39.3} \diagdown 7.160$

UA = WNL; PT/PTT = 12/25.1

g. *Blood:* T&C for 2 U PRBCs

h. *Pre-op orders:* Prep and shave abd, n.p.o. p MN, void on call to OR, 1 g Mandol IV on call to OR—written (this can also be abbreviated to simply: Pre-op orders—written)

Preoperative antibiotics will vary according to different surgeons, hospitals, and procedures, although many institutions are now developing standard protocols for certain surgeries, such as cholecystectomy or colectomy.

---

4. *Operative note:* You can write this if you went to the surgery. You will usually do so in the OR while the patient is being prepared for transport to the recovery room, or in the RR itself, while the resident is writing the postoperative orders.

   a. Pre-op Dx

   b. Procedure

   c. Post-op Dx

   d. Surgeon/ass'ts: (Put the names in order of rank with the attending surgeon first and yourself last.)

   e. Anesthesia: Local vs. general endotracheal (GET)

   f. *Findings:* This includes anything you found out about the patient during the procedure, such as frozen section results, stone in the common bile duct, metastatic studding of omentum or perineum, etc.

   g. *Specimen:* Whatever was removed from the patient's body and sent to pathology

   h. *Tubes/drains:* NGT, ETT, Foley, and especially drains from the wound area such as chest tubes, Penrose drains, Hemovac drains, etc. Be sure to specify how all these are being drained, e.g., NGT to low continuous wall suction; Foley to gravity drainage; chest tube to 15 cm of water suction or waterseal only on the Pleurovac, etc.

    i. *EBL:* The anesthesiologist can help you with this esti-
mate of blood loss

    j. *Fluids given:* Total of blood, crystalloid and colloid,
listed separately

    k. *Complications:* You don't want to know about these. If
there are any ask the resident how to word this section

    l. *Patient's condition and disposition:* Hopefully, the pa-
tient is transferred to the RR in stable condition

A more detailed operative summary will also need to be dictated. This summary will almost invariably be done by the resident or attending surgeon.

---

5. *Postoperative orders:* In most hosptitals, all previous orders
are voided on call to the OR, so you must now begin again
with a complete set of orders as if the patient were being
readmitted. This includes all the usual admission orders
plus:

    a. *IV:* You may want to include replacement for NG out-
put (usually ordered as ½ cc of ½ NS with 10 mEq of
KCl for each 1 cc of NG loss)

    b. *Diet:* Most patients will be n.p.o. If this will be neces-
sary for more than 3 to 5 days, you should consider PPN
or TPN. This decision will be influenced by the patient's preoperative nutritional status, the length of
time the patient is expected to be n.p.o., and the patient's catabolic state

---

In most recovery rooms there is a protocol for transferring patients to the ward when they are stable. If you have any special plans (such as sending the patient to the ICU), you'll need to specify these in the orders.

---

    c. *Chronic meds:* These can be a problem while the pa-
tient is n.p.o. Any solution must be individualized for

the particular patient. Essentially, eliminate whatever you can for the short term, give others IV if possible, change other required drugs to alternatives that can be given IV, and as a last resort, you may want to give elixir form meds via the NGT—clamp it for 1 hour and then release it

d. *Early ambulation:* This helps to reduce the risk of postop atelectasis and thrombophlebitis. OOB to chair is a first step toward ambulation that can generally be tolerated within 24 hours after even major surgery

e. *Pulmonary toilet:* This can include:
   (1) Turn, cough, and deep breathe (TC&DB) q1-2h
   (2) Chest PT q4-6h
   (3) Incentive spirometer to bedside; RN to instruct patient in its use
   (4) ETS (endotracheal suction) p.r.n.—only for patients who really can't cough by themselves
   (5) Trendelenburg x 1 hour q2-6h

How much you order in the way of pulmonary toilet will be determined by the patient's risk of pulmonary problems, but all patients who have had general anesthesia probably should TC&DB, and have an incentive spirometer at the bedside.

---

f. *Thromboembolic prophylaxis:* This may include leg elevation, TED hose, ace wraps to LEs, ASA, dextran, Persantine, or SQ heparin. Usually only leg elevation is used, unless the patient is at increased risk, such as with a previous history of DVT or with orthopedic procedures

g. *Tubes/drains:* Be sure to specify site and mode of drainage, as well as any tests to be done on the fluids (e.g., guaiac NG aspirate)

h. Due to void by 6 to 8 hours post-op (you'll be called if they don't)

  i. *Daily weights, I&Os:* Should be done for at least 48 hours to almost all patients because of the complexities of fluid management in the perioperative period

  j. *Wound care:* The standard order is: Leave operative dressing intact for 72 hours, then DSD (dry sterile dressing) q.d. and p.r.n. If the wound is being left open, you may want to have the nurses clean it with ¼% acetic-acid-soaked gauze (or any of several other solutions including sterile saline, Betadine, or half hydrogen peroxide and water). The wound can also then be packed with gauze soaked in one of these solutions, layered with two pieces of soaked mesh gauze, followed by layers of dry gauze, and then taped in place. This is called acetic acid (or saline, etc.) wet-to-dry dressings. Its advantage is that it tends to autodebride the wound when the dressing is changed

  k. *Post-op labs:* As indicated by specific circumstances

  l. *Meds:* Must include adequate analgesia. Initial order should be for smaller doses q3–4h. Too much narcotic will cause respiratory suppression, and too much pain will lead to hypoventilation because of splinting. Tailor this individually, based on the patient's size, relative risks, and narcotic use. A good starting point for a 70 kg patient is 50 to 100 mg IM Demerol with 25 to 50 mg of IM Phenergan or Vistaril (the former is more effective at combatting nausea but is a narcotic antagonist, the latter is a narcotic agonist). The range is given so the nurses can assess the patient's individual needs and response to narcotics

  m. *Panic orders:* VS limits for which you want to be called

6. *Postoperative check:* This can be written in the usual SOAP format:

  • **S:** Be sure to include history of voiding since the OR (unless the patient has a Foley), respiratory c/os, and c/os of pain suggestive of inadequate analgesia

- **O:** I&Os since OR
  The PE should always include VS, mental status, heart, lungs, abdomen, extremities (especially for signs of DVT), dressing (you don't need to examine the wound directly unless the dressing is soaked with drainage)
  Labs Since OR
- **AP:** Stable—routine post-op care (or more as indicated)

7. *Postoperative fever evaluation:* Remember the 5 Ws

A low-grade fever in the first 24 hours post-op doesn't usually merit a work-up, unless the patient appears to be more ill than would be expected. Such fever is almost certainly caused by atelectasis.

- Wind: Early as atelectasis, later as pneumonia
- Walking: Either DVT or its sequela, pulmonary embolus
- Wonder Drug: As in drug reaction
- Water: As in UTI
- Wound: As in infection or even abscess formation
  The second and third Ws can occur at any time during the post-op course. Atelectasis is always the most likely explanation, and in the first 24 hours post-op, it accounts for more than 95% of all fevers. UTI is most likely to occur two or more days after Foley insertion. Wound infection is unlikely to occur before 3 to 5 days post-op.

8. *Procedures*
   a. *Cutting sutures:* This is the main responsibility of a scutboy in the OR. You will be shown how to hold the scissors. The surgeon will often show you how far from the knot to cut the suture, but you'll be ahead of the game if you have a general idea. The length of tie left with the knot is somewhat subjective, and also dependent on where the suture is (SQ should be cut shorter than perineal or fascial ties).

- Short (1 to 2 mm): Silk or braided materials
- Medium (3 to 4 mm): Chromic and gut
- Long (5 to 6 mm): Monofilament synthetic materials (nylon, Prolene, etc.)

As the name implies, absorbable sutures will be absorbed and do not generally need to be removed. These include natural materials (gut) and synthetic materials (Dexon, Vicryl). Nonabsorbable sutures include nylon, dacron, and Prolene. The diameter of the suture material is noted by a number of "zeros" (e.g., 4-0, 5-0). The finer the thread, the more zeros.

---

b. *Staple placement and removal:* The use of staples has decreased the opportunities for scutboys to learn how to suture skin, which is unfortunate. You will usually staple the skin while the resident everts the edges. Place the stapler right next to the forceps on the skin, staple, and slide the stapler forward off the now imbedded staple. To remove staples, tell the patient it won't hurt much, look confident, and be as quick as possible without pulling at the skin. If the wound edges start to separate, stop and check with your resident. Often the solution is to apply the tapes between the staples before removing the latter. If you are concerned about a wound opening, you can remove alternating staples initially and look for problems.

Usually staples are removed between 5 to 7 days post-op. Some surgeons like to remove the staples before the patient leaves the hospital, others use it as a reason for seeing the patient within the first few days after discharge.

---

c. *Surgical tapes (e.g., Steri-Strips):* Generally, every patient will get Steri-Strips after suture removal. Clean the skin surrounding the wound, dry it carefully, and apply benzoin tincture compound on both sides of the wound. If you're using an aerosol, cover the wound with a 4 x 4 gauze before spraying on the benzoin. Let the benzoin dry, at which point it will be extremely sticky (this is to help the tapes adhere). Then peel the tapes and apply them across the wound. This can be done neatly and quickly by applying the leading edge of a whole card of tapes to one side of the wound and then peeling the card away while pressing the tapes in place. Some people cut the tapes in half before applying them, both for aesthetic and economic reasons. Tell the patients that after 24 hours they can wash as if the tapes weren't there, and that the tapes will gradually fall off by themselves over the following 2 weeks. The patient should never peel the tapes off, because they can pull their wound open trying to remove a very adherent tape.

Tapes are most often used to ensure wound closure after sutures or, more commonly, staples have been removed. In some institutions tapes are also used to close small traumatic wounds, especially on children.

M. OBSTETRICS AND GYNECOLOGY ROTATION
Mark W. Woodruff

First, a word about gynecology is in order. As a surgically oriented subspecialty, the scut of inpatient gynecology differs very little from the principles outlined in the previous section. One main difference to remember is the need to include the patient's gynecologic history in the initial paragraph of your H&P. This information should include the patient's parity, age at menarche and menopause, last menstrual period (the date of the first day of the LMP, by convention) and menstrual pattern (frequency, regularity, length of bleeding and an estimate of amount in number of pads or tampons per day, any history of midcycle bleeding, and any difficulties in the past), birth control method presently used and any others used in the past, previous gynecologic surgery, and family history of relevant cancers if the patient is being evaluated for cancer. Other than that, this rotation isn't much different from being on the general surgery service, except all the patients are female.

In gynecologic clinics, you will see many problems, often unrelated to gynecology. Foremost among the complaints presenting to an outpatient gynecology clinic are the need for birth control, routine health maintenance (breast and pelvic exams and Pap smear), lower abdominal pain (often not gynecologic in origin), and abnormal vaginal bleeding. These problems are beyond the scope of this book, but you can read about them in any standard gynecologic textbook.

Obstetrics can be one of the most exciting, pleasant, and rewarding rotations you do, but for many of us, it is also quite frightening. It is usually the closest any medical student comes to being responsible in an "emergency" situation, defined as one in which things are happening too quickly for you to go back to your book bag to look something up in that spiral-bound manual you bought. If you're going to deliver a baby, which most medical students do, you'll have to be prepared to react almost automatically. That's difficult when you're doing something for the first time, but you should have the resident right behind you. The best way to reduce anxiety is to make an index card with the steps of delivery on it and review it frequently until it becomes second nature.

It may sound corny, but be sure to allow yourself to stop and appreciate the significance of what you're seeing, to look at it from a personal, rather then medical, viewpoint. You may be surprised by what you see.

In the midst of all that activity, its worthwhile to remember two things: First, this is a natural process in which you participate, not a procedure that you do to someone. It would most likely all turn out fine without you even being there. Second, for mother and child (and, it is hoped, father as well), this is a very significant personal moment in their lives. Anything you can do to facilitate their experience is a real service.

1. *Admission history and physical examination:* This should be briefer and more focused than any other H&P you'll do, partly by virtue of time constraints (sometimes they're wheeling the patient directly from the admitting office to the delivery room) and also by the nature of the patient—a young, generally healthy person who isn't really *ill* at all.

   Different formats can be used, but this is the information you'll need to include:

   Jane Doe is a 29 yo WF, G_3 P_{2002}, LMP 12/15, EDC (estimated date of confinement, or due date) by dates 9/21. New OB exam at 11 weeks EGA (estimated gestational age) and U/S (ultrasound exam) at 20 weeks EGA were consistent with dates. She is now $39\frac{1}{2}$ weeks EGA. Tonight she noted the gradual onset of increasingly strong contractions. During the last hour they were every 4 minutes, lasting approximately 1 minute and moderately strong with pain in her back as well as her abdomen. She denies recent fever, vaginal bleeding, or SROM (spontaneous rupture of membranes, heralded by a liter or more of fluid exiting rapidly from the patient's vagina). She's been on prenatal vitamins and iron pills throughout her pregnancy and her prenatal course has otherwise been remarkable only for two UTIs.

Parity is abbreviated as follows: P_{1234}
   1 = Full-term deliveries
   2 = Premature deliveries (between 20 and 37 weeks EGA)
   3 = Abortions (spontaneous and elective aren't distinguished)
   4 = Living children at present
The mnemonic for this is *Florida Power And Light.*

Her prenatal screening lab work is as follows: 0+ blood type; RPR-NR; GC culture–negative; pap smear–Class I; rubella immune; Hct = 34% (generally known as the Big 6).

a. *Past obstetrical history:* This can most easily be set up in a tabular format, as follows:

Dates	Outcome (AB, NSVD, etc.)	Sex	Weight	Length of Labor	Complications/ Problems

b. *PMH:* If she's had any major medical problems
c. *Social history:* If this may affect delivery or the baby's care, i.e., if the mother has poor social supports

---

A summary of the history is: age/parity/LMP/EDC/EGA/present labor/prenatal course/present meds/Big 6/Past OB Hx/PMH/SH (if relevant).

---

d. *PE:* Should include VS, a brief HEENT exam, heart and lungs, abdominal exam including FH (fundal height), FHT (fetal heart tones), the presenting part of the baby (vertex: head down; breech: buttocks down), pelvic exam (describe cervical effacement, dilation, and baby's presentation, position, and station), and extremities exam (reflexes and edema), plus any other specifically relevant exam.

The nomenclature for the baby's orientation can be confusing, but it is simply described as follows:
  (a) Lie is the relationship of the long axis of the baby to that of the mother (i.e., transverse, longitudinal, or oblique)
  (b) Presentation refers to the part presenting itself at the pelvic inlet (e.g., breech, vertex, or mentum presentation)
  (c) Position refers to the direction the baby is facing (ROA, ROP, etc.)
  (d) The baby's station is the progress of the presenting part through the birth canal (e.g., +1, 0 or −1)

If the patient has been there long enough to have a tracing on the external fetal monitor (EFM), you should also describe it, giving particular attention to the character of the mother's contractions, any decelerations of the fetal heart rate, and looking for adequate elevation of the fetal heart rate with activity (also known as an FAT or fetal activity test).

    e. *Assessment and plan:* Term IUP; active labor
       (1) EFM
       (2) Routine labor room care and admitting lab work
       (3) Follow labor expectantly, vaginal delivery anticipated

2. *Admission orders*
    a. Admit to Labor and Delivery
    b. *Dx:* Term IUP, active labor
    c. *Condition:* Stable
    e. *VS:* Per routine
    e. *Activity:* Bedrest after enema
    f. *Diet:* N.P.O.
    g. *Labs:* UA, CBC, hold clot (in some hospitals an RPR is also done)
    h. EFM
    i. Prep and shave perineum
    j. Fleet enema now

Shaving the perineum and giving an enema are very controversial. The former is intended mainly to improve sterile conditions during delivery (a contradiction in terms), and to make the delivery easier for the physician. There are many arguments for giving an enema: it's easier for the patient to go to the bathroom during early labor than late labor; it decreases contamination during delivery; it decreases "fecal dystocia"; it's embarrassing for some patients to defecate during delivery, which may cause them to hold back instead of pushing; and it's nicer for the physician. The arguments against are that it's uncomfortable for the patient and it's another example of unnecessary and intrusive actions by the physician into a natural process. A reasonable compromise is to shave or clip only the bottom half of the perineum (not the mons) and give a single Fleet enema. Make sure you do the pelvic exam first—an enema is contraindicated in a patient who is near complete dilation, for obvious reasons.

NB: This list does not include a standing order for analgesic, which in most cases you will want to order specifically as the labor progresses.

Obstetrical nurses are more involved in the patient's care and generally more resistant to residents and students than any other group of nurses, largely because in many settings they function somewhat like residents. They do most of the things the doctor does, including deliver the baby if there's no doctor there in time (remember—tide, time, and a multiparous female wait for no one). The best way to get along with them as a medical student is to be respectful, learn as much as you can from them, and otherwise stay out of their way.

---

3. *Managing labor:* Though this sounds more like a business school topic, it is one of the most challenging parts of obstetrical care. Fortunately, the residents and nurses will do most of it. There are a few general principles to keep in mind: (a) analgesia is important, but too much systemic analgesic too early can slow or halt even real labor. Other options include spinal or epidural blocks and pudendal blocks; (b) frequent exams are generally unnecessary, especially in primiparous patients. Every 1 to 3 hours is perfectly adequate unless she has the urge to push; (c) it's advisable to sit with one or two patients through their labor, to get a better idea of what the woman experiences. If the patient has no labor coach, you can fill that gap.

The main things a labor coach tries to provide are: (a) a calming influence; (b) reminders to conserve energy by not "fighting" the contractions—i.e., don't tense the whole body with each contraction; (c) physical comforting—rubbing the back, or whatever makes the woman feel better, and (d) someone to yell at during transition. Don't take personally whatever the woman says—Bill Cosby's wife reputedly told the whole delivery ward that his parents weren't married. If you get a chance to act as a labor coach, take it. It will give you a different perspective on the birth process.

4. *Delivery:* The important principles to remember are that the baby will generally be born on its own, but that you can augment the process and help protect the mother from some of the bad sequelae of childbirth, principally perineal stretching and pelvic relaxation. You can also help the woman by being a cheerleader. Often she is tired when the time for delivery comes, and needs a little help to mount the effort to successfully deliver her baby. You, along with the nurses and father, can provide that help. Learning how to best encourage each patient is a lifetime project, but the best way to start is by spending time with the patient during her labor and getting to know her.

   You will generally be delivering multiparous patients, so you will have an easier time, although probably less time. Make sure the resident attends all your deliveries, both so you will feel more secure and so he or she can teach you something.

Summary of Delivery:
- Prep yourself.
- Prep the patient.
- Deliver the head (with or w/o episiotomy).
- Suction nares and mouth and check for nuchal cords.
- Deliver the shoulders (A, then P).
- Deliver the body.
- Clamp and cut the cord.
- Pass the baby to the nurses.
- Deliver the placenta.
- Find and repair lacerations or episiotomy.

---

a. Scrub (2 to 3 minutes generally, less if the birth is imminent).
b. Gown and glove (sometimes done after prepping the patient).
c. Prep the patient (often done by the nurses).
d. Drape the patient (bottom sheet, two leg covers, and top sheet over the abdomen).
e. Check the baby's position by feeling the fontanelles (ROA, ROT, etc.). At this point you would put in the pudendal block if you were going to use this method of anesthesia.

This is where it is very helpful to have your instruments laid out well and close at hand, because you don't want to look away from the baby if at all possible, and you should not under any circumstances take your hand off the baby's head. The next contraction could be the one to finish the birth.

---

f. Set up your table and wheel it closer to you for better access. Lay out the instruments in the order of use during delivery: suction bulb, two clamps for cord, scissors; you can worry about sutures later.
g. Consider cutting an episiotomy. This is another controversy in obstetrics.

In many multiparous patients, an episiotomy is clearly needless surgery. You can read about the types and modes of repair in any textbook. There are several key points to remember: (a) before you cut, achieve adequate anesthesia with an SQ injection of a local anesthetic (usually 1% lidocaine with epinephrine); (b) cut when the baby is beginning to stretch the introitus (when 3 to 4 cm of head is visible with each contraction), and (c) cut inward more than downward to maximize the benefit if your incision.

If you don't cut an episiotomy, make sure you keep the perineum and introitus moist with wet 4 x 4s and prepare the perineum by stretching the birth canal with two fingers on each side just ahead of the baby's head, working the tissue back over the head as it advances.

h. As you encourage the mother to push with each contraction, more and more of the head will emerge. As you deliver the head, four principles should be remembered:

(1) The head in the usual OA position is delivered in a J-type motion, moving deeply posteriorly (toward the rectum), then coming anteriorly by extension of the neck after the BPD (biparietal diameter) reaches the vulva.

(2) Most perineal damage, both in terms of stretching and lacerations, is caused by rapid expulsion of the baby's head. You are encouraging the mother to push the baby out, but with your left hand you should be holding the top of the head so you can control the rate of expulsion in its final moments.

(3) Cover your right hand with a towel, and place it on the perineum just posterior to the introitus; pressure here on the chin will help deliver the head as the neck extends.

(4) The mother should be pushing only with contractions, when she has the full benefit of the uterine force to help her; in between contractions she should rest, and you should massage and moisten the perineum.

i. The rest of the action generally (unless there is shoulder dystocia) goes very quickly, so you need to be prepared. As soon as the head is delivered, tell the mother to stop pushing, and keep your left hand on the baby's head in case the mother fails to follow instructions. With your right hand, run your fingertips from the baby's ear to the shoulder to check for nuchal cord loops. If one is present clear it posterior to anterior (you can stretch fairly hard). If it can't be cleared, clamp and cut the cord and deliver the baby immediately.

Again with your right hand, grab the bulb syringe and suction both nostrils and the mouth (pointing the tip laterally rather than straight back in the mouth).

j. You now want to deliver the shoulders, but first you must move them from a coronal to a sagittal orientation. Usually the baby will rotate by itself, but you can help by putting your hands over each ear with your fingers extending as far as possible down on the shoulders, and gently turning the baby in whichever direction shows less resistance. This will generally be toward the original orientation of the baby (remember ROA).

Next, you must deliver the anterior shoulder, followed by the posterior. This requires strength and control. The objective is to move the entire body posteriorly so the anterior shoulder can move past the pubic bone. The trick is to do it without bending or stressing the cervical spine. Position your hands as above and move the body posteriorly with slow steady pressure until the anterior shoulder pops out, then move the body anteriorly until the posterior shoulder is delivered.

k. At this point the body will most likely slide right out; if not, you can hook a thumb and index finger in each axilla and pull the baby out. The baby will be wet and slippery. It's considered poor form to drop the object of all this time and effort, yet it's easy to do. The best way to avoid this faux pas is the cradle the baby to your body. Make sure you support the head. Clamp the cord in two places and cut it in between the clamps. Pass the baby to the nurse or put it under the warmer yourself. The nurses will generally take care of the baby from this point.

By holding the baby below the level of the uterus, you can give it a small autotransfusion from the placenta. This can be accomplished by bending your knees while you're suctioning the baby and clamping the cord, or it can occur automatically if you have the delivery bed raised to the level of your axilla before delivery, and then hold the baby at waist height.

l. Return to the mother. Firmly massage the uterine fundus to encourage adequate and continued contraction (the main mechanism of bleeding control). If bleeding is severe, you may need to manually extract the placenta and massage the uterus intravaginally as well as abdominally. At this point, you should also draw blood from the cord according to hospital protocol. The nurses will generally tell you how much to draw and have everything laid out for you. It is generally a good idea to draw 10 to 20 cc on the baby of any Rh negative mother. Some hospitals do Hct and blood type with direct Coomb's test on cord blood from all babies.

m. Move your clamp up the remaining cord and then apply mild, steady tension on the cord to help with the placental delivery. When pulling on the cord, don't press on the top of the fundus, or you may evert the uterus, which is also frowned upon in most circles. You can press downward just over the pubic bone.

You are never supposed to pull on the cord until the placenta has separated from the wall of the uterus, but this is often difficult to determine in practice.

Delivery of the placenta may take up to 5 to 10 minutes. If it is approaching this time limit (some physicians will wait slightly longer), you or the resident may choose to reach into the uterus and manually extract the placenta. The major concern here is to avoid everting the uterus.

As the placenta delivers, twist it to help get all of the membranes, which will follow the placenta out. It may be helpful to take hold of the membranes with a ring forceps to help get all of them. Retained placental material will increase the risk of postpartum hemorrhage.

Be sure to examine the placenta for spaces, indicative of material retained in the uterus. Check the cord for three vessels—two arteries and one large vein.

After the placenta is delivered, the patient should receive oxytocin to help the uterus contract and thus control bleeding. This can be given IV (if the patient has one) or IM. Usually a total dose of 10 to 20 U is given, or 1 to 2 ml of the usual oxytocin solution. This can be given as a bolus IM or over 5 to 10 minutes by IV.

n. Inspect the cervix and the rest of the birth canal for lacerations. The easiest way to do this is to put a 4 x 4 gauze in a ring forceps, put this in the vagina and lift anteriorly (to hold the bladder out of the way), while placing two fingers in the vagina and pressing down posteriorly. This should expose the cervix for inspection. You may have to take hold of the anterior lip of the cervix with the clamp to adequately see the posterior portion. Lacerations of 2 cm or less will generally heal spontaneously without any repair. Any cervical laceration associated with excessive postpartum bleeding is more worrisome, as this may be the source of the bleeding. Be sure to examine the rest of the birth canal, including the periurethral area. Lacerations here can be repaired with a few interrupted sutures, just to reoppose the mucosal edges and thereby speed the healing process.

o. Assuming the bleeding has slowed, you can now close the episiotomy and repair any perineal lacerations. This may require more local anesthesia even if you gave some before cutting the episiotomy. The tissue near the anus is by far the most sensitive, so give extra anesthetic here. The best way to learn how to close an episiotomy is to watch several and then have someone walk you through you first one step by step. The anatomy can be difficult to visualize correctly. Fortunately, most any repair will give an adequate result. The repair can be done with any 2-0 or 3-0 absorbable suture material. Remember that postpartum discomfort will be directly related to the number of knots you leave, so a subcuticular perineal closure is best (see any standard textbook for further details). The main goals are to reapproximate the edges of the hymeneal ring remnant and to close the mucosa.

5. *Delivery note:* Now the paperwork begins. This will vary, but there are often several forms (including the labor and delivery record and the birth certificate) that need to be completed and signed, usually by the resident. You can write the delivery note:
   a. *Dx:* Term IUP
   b. *Procedure:* NSVD
   c. *Obstetrician:* Your name/resident's name
   d. *Anesthesia:* Local (or whatever type of block was used; analgesia doesn't need to be listed here)
   e. *Episiotomy/lacerations:* Midline episiotomy, no lacerations, repaired with 3-0 prolene
   f. *Findings:* Term female, 7 lb, 8 oz, Apgars 8/9, placenta intact with three vessel cord
   g. *EBL:* 400 cc
   h. *Complications:* None
   i. Mother to recovery; baby to newborn nursery in good condition

6. *Postpartum orders*
   a. Admit to PP ward

    b. *Dx:* S/P NSVD

    c. *VSs:* Per routine

    d. *Activity:* OOB with assistance first 12 hours, 10 ad lib

    e. *Perineal care:* Ice pack PP p.r.n.

    f. *Episiotomy care:* Perineal lamp b.i.d. p.r.n., start 12 hours PP, hot sitz baths t.i.d. p.r.n., Methergine 0.2 mg p.o. q4h × 6 doses

    g. *Pain med:* Take your choice, usually Tylenol No. 3 with NSVD, IM Demerol and Phenergan with C-sections

    h. *Sleeping med:* Take your choice (avoid in breast-feeding moms)

    i. *Laxative:* Of choice

    j. *Feeding:* Breast or bottle

    k. *Breast care* (if bottle feeding): Breast binders, ice packs p.r.n.; consider Parlodel 2.5 mg p.o. b.i.d. with meals 14 days

    l. *Rh Immune globulin:* If mom is Rh negative and baby Rh positive

    m. Complete admission lab work (sometimes there isn't time to get a urine specimen between admission and delivery).

7. *Postpartum care:* Round on your patients daily, checking how the patients are feeling, for progressive slowing of their bleeding and vaginal discharge (lochia), how they're doing with their new baby in terms of feeding and bonding, and any s/syx of postpartum complications. You should palpate the fundus to make sure it's remained firm and is decreasing in size. A brief note will suffice.

8. *Discharge instructions:* When the patient is ready to go home, you need to anticipate her problems and questions. This will help allay her fears and also decrease follow-up phone calls later. The following topics should be covered, as well as any questions she already has.

Generally, you can refer any questions about the baby to the pediatrician, who should also be seeing the mother every day and giving her discharge instructions and advice about the baby.

She should continue her prenatal vitamins if breast-feeding, and iron sulfate if indicated for anemia. Other medicines if they're indicated, particularly a pain medicine, usually Tylenol No. 3 or Percocet if she is S/P C-section.

Breast binders or a tight-fitting bra and a prescription for Parlodel (if you choose to use it) are indicated for discomfort if mother isn't breast-feeding. Breast-feeding mothers should be instructed to keep their nipple dry between feedings, and to use Vitamin E oil or lanolin when the inevitable nipple discomfort begins. You can also reassure them that this problem is generally self-limited and does not require stopping breast-feeding to resolve.

She can continue sitz baths to help with perineal discomfort. She can resume sexual activity whenever she feels comfortable, but most patients wait at least 2 or 3 weeks. She needs to know that she can get pregnant without having a period first. Her period may return anytime from 2 weeks PP to 1 year or more if she's breast-feeding. Breast-feeding mothers need to be reminded that this isn't adequate birth control. Her lochia will diminish and stop completely over the ensuing 1 to 2 weeks.

It is normal to have some emotional letdown during the weeks following the "big event," even including some crying spells. If this gets severe enough to interfere with your patient's ability to care for or bond with the baby, she needs to call the doctor's office right away.

She will need to be seen for a follow-up evaluation and examination approximately 6 weeks after the baby is born.

9. *OB-GYN clinic:* The purpose of these visits is to check for adequate progression of the pregnancy, screen for potential

complications of pregnancy, and assist the mother in adjusting to her pregnancy and preparing for childbirth. The anticipatory guidance you give is as important as the exam. Most clinics will have a flow sheet, hopefully covering all three of the above areas. A minimum clinic visit should include:

a. *Hx:* Quickening (the mother's sensation of fetal movement)—include any change in frequency; Hx of edema; other issues relevant to the particular trimester (such as N&V in the first, birth classes in the second, and contractions or fluid leak in the third trimester)

b. *Physical exam:* Should include BP, edema, FH, FHT (note whether they were heard with doppler or fetoscope), fetal position (third trimester), and cervix check (after 37 weeks)

c. *Labs:* Most clinics check the urine at every visit for protein and glucose, although there's no conclusive evidence this is necessary. Other screening tests will be needed at various times throughout the pregnancy, such as the Big 6 at the initial visit and the glucola or O'Sullivan screen for diabetes at 26 weeks

d. *AP:* Assuming everything is going well, patients will return to the clinic: every 4 weeks until 28 weeks; every 2 weeks until 36 weeks; weekly until delivery

10. *Six-week check:* The relevant history at this visit includes confirming the lochia stopping, any history of menses, sexual activity, and birth control use. It's also nice to ask how the baby is doing.

Generally, a brief physical exam (heart, lungs, etc.) is done in addition to a pelvic exam and pap smear. You should make sure they have an adequate form of birth control (fit them for a diaphragm, prescribe OCPs etc.), and remind them to return in 1 year for their routine screening Pap smear and pelvic exam.

N. PEDIATRICS ROTATION
Mark W. Woodruff

Inpatient pediatrics involves a broad range of activities, varying with the setting, such as newborn nursery, intensive care nursery, and the pediatric ward. It is hoped that you will also get some exposure to an outpatient clinic, as this is the bulk of pediatric practice.

One must remember with all pediatric patients that a special level of sensitivity is needed, as they often don't understand what's going on and are not as capable of dealing with their fears as most adult patients. In addition, the traditional doctor–patient dyad is expanded to a triad with the inclusion of the parent(s). You will learn much about the fine art of negotiation in this context.

The main principles of initial neonatal care in the delivery room are to keep the baby warm by drying it off and putting it under a warmer, and to stimulate the baby enough to encourage adequate respirations. If stimulation isn't doing the job, or there are other indications of problems, then it is a "code" situation and the ABCDs (airway, breathing, cardiovascular, drugs) come into play.

---

1. *Delivery room:* A pediatrician is generally present at all C-sections, meconium or premature deliveries, or when problems are anticipated. If you go, your main role will be to help assign Apgar scores. They are assigned at 1, 5, and sometimes 10 minutes, and are intended to signify risk of neonatal complications. Only the 5 and 10 minutes scores have been shown to have significant predictive value. The scores are somewhat subjective, but the official guidelines are shown on the following page.

2. *Newborn physical examination:* You can't adequately learn about this exam or most other medicine just by reading. Most nurseries will have a standard form you will need to

	Apgar Score		
	0	1	2
Color	Blue, pale	Body pink, extremities blue	All pink
Muscle tone	Flaccid	Some extremity flexion	Good flexion, active motion
Respirations	Absent	slow, irregular	Regular, crying
Heart rate	Absent	< 100	> 100
Reflex irritability (to nasal suctioning)	No response	Grimace	Vigorous cry

complete. Babies generally get a complete physical exam on admission and again at discharge, as well as standard screening blood work done by state labs, the results of which you'll never see.

If you spend part of your rotation in the newborn nursery, take advantage of the opportunity by feeding, rocking, and holding some of the babies. It will help break down any barriers you may have in dealing with them and also help you to be more understanding with the parents. It won't hurt if you ever have any children of your own, either.

The physical exam should be done with the baby completely naked. You'll need a tape measure, ophthalmoscope, stethoscope, tongue depressor, and diaper. You should wash you hands thoroughly before examining any baby and most nurseries also require that you wear a gown over your clothes. Remember, the main thing you're looking for is congenital anomalies.

  a. *General appearance:* You can comment on muscle tone (how much resistance and return flexion there is to extending the arms), cry, color, and edema

b. *Skin:* Particularly focusing on any lesions, cyanosis, or jaundice (which generally starts on the head and movers caudally)

c. *Head/neck:* Describe any molding (irregular shape of the skull from prolonged labor), cephalhematoma (subperiosteal hematoma, usually tense, nonmobile and always with definable edges near the edges of cranial bone(s)), and caput succedaneum (subcutaneous hematoma or fluid collection, distinguished from cephalhematoma by being softer, mobile, not following cranial suture lines and reabsorbing within hours to days)

d. *Eyes:* Look through the ophthalmoscope and see the "red" reflex, which is often white, but shows there's a retina and a clear path for light to reach it. Make sure your hands and the baby's eyes are dry before trying to pry its lids open

e. *Ears, nose, and throat:* Make sure the ear canals are patent, the palate is intact (feel it with your finger and check the suck reflex at the same time) and look at the pharynx and uvula (bifid uvula is a clue to incomplete palate fusion)

f. *Thorax:* Feel the breasts on boys and girls, they'll generally contain 1 to 2 cm of palpable breast tissue. If this is absent, it's a suggestion of prematurity

g. *Lungs*

h. *Cardiovascular:* Listen to the heart and feel the femoral pulses

i. *Abdomen:* Assuming the appearance is normal, you're mainly feeling for masses; this requires deep palpation of both sides of the abdomen with the fingers of one hand while the other hand supports the back on the side being palpated

j. *Genitalia:* Females will often have a discharge, sometimes bloody, because of withdrawal of maternal estrogen. Make sure both testes are down in males. You will not be able to retract the foreskin, so don't try

k. *Anus:* You can usually ascertain patency by visual inspection alone

l. *Trunk and spine:* Check for gross abnormalities. Careful attention needs to be paid to the skin overlying the spine for subtle sinus tracts indicating incomplete fusion of the spine

m. *Extremities:* Carefully palpate over the clavicles for crepitus, indicative of a fracture sustained during delivery. You also need to manipulate the hips to check for possible congenital dislocation. Ortolani's sign is a palpable click when abducting the flexed hip. It requires an orthopedic referral if the hip remains in the dislocated position. A tendency to dislocate can sometimes be treated successfully with triple diapering. You should also check carefully for extra digits. These will often be vestigial in appearance with only a small skin tag on the ulnar aspect of the hand or fifth finger

n. *Reflexes:* Normal reflexes in the neonate include plantar and palmar grasp (elicited by placing your finger on the baby's sole or palm), suck in response to anything resembling a nipple put in the mouth, and the Moro reflex. The Moro reflex is elicited by grasping the infant's hands and extending and abducting the arms sufficiently to raise the shoulders but not the head off the crib, and then releasing, which should cause an embracing response. A normal Moro reflex brings both arms across the midline

3. *Admission history and physical examination:* This differs very little from a work-up on the medicine rotation, except the history is shorter. In infants less than 1 year of age, the first paragraph of the HPI should include the mother's prenatal course and the baby's neonatal history including birth weight and length and any complications of delivery. With all children the SH is very important and should

include who lives in the home, who cares for the child, any disruptions at home, siblings, and school performance including grades repeated if applicable. It is acceptable to comment on the family interactions (as you saw them) in the general section of the physical exam.

An admission physical exam should be complete from head to toe. The order of examination in an infant is different than in an adult, however. You must first listen to the heart and lungs, hopefully before the child starts crying. If the child is still cooperative, proceed with the abdominal and extremities exam. The HEENT exam should generally be done last, with the understanding that screaming can cause engorgement of the vessels of the TM leading to the appearance of otitis media, in which case added weight must be put on eardrum mobility with insufflation. A normal eardrum will flutter, whereas a drum with serous fluid behind it will move stiffly or not at all.

You may want to examine the child with or without the parents present, with the parent either holding the baby or standing next to the baby while the baby is on the examining table or bed. Overall, I believe the best way is to have the infant on the parent's lap. In this method the exam is done in the order described above with the exception of the abdominal exam, which requires the patient to be supine and therefore is done last. For the HEENT exam, the child is held facing you, with the parent's leg crossed over both of the child's legs, one of the parent's arms around the child's arms and body and the other arm around the child's head. This technique has the advantage that the child is with the parent (presumably feeling more secure) and that the parent, not you, is restraining the child.

As a medical student, however, it may be easier for you not to have the parent(s) present as you work your way through the exam. In this case one person can immobilize an infant for otoscopic exam in the following manner: The child is placed face down on the exam table with hands at its sides (if you have an assistant, that person can hold both the child's hands stretched over the child's head). You lay your chest over the child's back, pinning the arm closest to you with your body and the other arm is held down with your right upper arm. You still have both hands free. With the butt of your left hand, you will hold the child's head in place, while the last three fingers hold the insufflation bulb, and the index finger and thumb pull back on the pinna to straighten the ear canal. Your right hand manipulates the otoscope. This procedure is a delicate amalgam of several methods commonly used on the professional wrestling circuit and is guaranteed to do the job.

Distracting the patient during the physical exam is generally overrated, but can sometimes be helpful. This is why pediatricians have little stuffed animals on their stethoscopes and decal pictures of animals on their beepers (at least the residents). A child's favorite toy can also be useful, but none of these can substitute for speed.

---

4. *Procedures*
    a. *Blood drawing:* The procedure is essentially the same as in adults, except for the crying, which can be unnerving. In infants and neonates, you'll use a 23- or 25-gauge butterfly, and remember to use pediatric-sized blood containers, commonly called bullets. Be careful to apply very little vacuum in drawing the blood, as there is more risk of vein collapse here than in adults. A good venipuncture will cause blood to flow down the butterfly without any vacuum; when the blood nears the end of the tubing, an assistant should attach the syringe and apply 0.5 cc of vacuum.

    Leg veins are acceptable targets. Use a rubber band for a tourniquet in infants. Blind attempts at a brachial vein are also acceptable, but should probably be performed by the resident. Remember, you can almost always get arterial blood, and this is an acceptable alternative if necessary.

b. *Arterial blood drawing:* Again, this is very similar to ABGs in adults. You may use a 21- or 23-gauge butterfly, and first perform a modified Allen test (squeeze the hand while compressing both the radial and ulnar arteries, then release the ulnar to assess its ability to supply the hand; the entire hand should pink up before you release the radial artery).

It is best to quickly insert the needle all the way in and then slowly withdraw it, watching for blood return. In an infant the return won't necessarily be pulsatile, but is should flow well. Make sure you aren't cutting off blood flow as you steady the arm. When making repeated attempts, you may occasionally feel as if you're in the artery in spite of a lack of blood return. This may be caused by old blood in the needle or hub clotting off, in which case you need a new butterfly. This clotting problem occurs even more easily with venipuncture, and is the reason why you should have several butterflies available before you start either procedure.

c. *Intravenous line placement:* Get everything prepared in advance, especially all your pieces of tape. In addition to the usual materials, you'll need an armboard for an IV in almost any patient under 18 yo. For infants and small children you'll also need something to cover the IV, such as an inverted 30 cc medicine cup with a V-section cut out for the hub of the IV to exit. A 3-cc syringe should be filled with sterile saline or water "flush" and attached to a T-connector (an insertible hub with a short piece of tubing coming off the side). You may find it easier to tape the child's arm to the armboard for better control before inserting the IV, but this results in a lot of extra work if you "blow" the vein.

In infants, a rubber band can be used as a tourniquet. Rubbing an alcohol wipe over the chosen site may be helpful. Don't forget the foot and ankle as potential IV sites. They are done essentially the same as an arm IV, the leg is anchored to a board, and then the leg is well wrapped with gauze to protect the IV if the child is active.

The angiocath size you use will vary depending on the size of the patient. Angiocaths are available as small as 24 gauge—the size most commonly used on infants and neonates.

As you try to thread the vein, advance slowly, stopping frequently to check for blood return. It may be slow, so watch for it in the catheter, not in the hub. Once you have entered the vein, advance slightly, then remove the needle and attach the flush. If slow injection of fluid doesn't raise a lump, you're probably in the vein. Advance the catheter gently to the hub and anchor it with your first pieces of tape. Tape the arm or leg to the board, putting gauze over the portion of tape to go over the arm, so you won't have to worry about skin damage later. Tape the four fingers over the end of the board and the thumb separately over the side. As you work, continue to flush periodically with 0.5 cc to maintain patency. When the arm is secure, connect the IV set. Cover the IV so only enough of the port is visible to wipe it off and inject any IV medications. Check the fingers to make sure all your taping hasn't hampered blood flow to the hand.

Avoid scalp vein IVs at all costs. They can cause nasty problems if they infiltrate, and it's possible to unknowingly catheterize a small artery, which can be dangerous if you're giving antibiotics through the IV. If they must be done, they should probably be done by the resident.

---

d. *Lumbar puncture:* This differs very little from performing an LP on an adult, except that it is usually significantly easier to enter the interspace. In an infant, make sure the child is well-flexed, but not so flexed as to interfere with his respiratory efforts. Proceed as in an adult, with the same approach to the anatomy (L4–5 or L3–4 interspace, parallel with the top of the iliac crests). The angle of the insertion is closer to 90° in an infant than in an adult, but is still directed somewhat cephalad. Remember the dimensions are reduced, so you won't need to go too deep. Withdraw the stylet frequently as you advance. It is not customary to measure opening pressures in children. Collect at least 0.5 cc in each tube. After completing the LP, make sure there isn't a CSF leak before you put a bandage over the needle insertion site.

SECTION 2

The Practice of Scut

A. GRAM'S STAIN

The ability to make a good Gram's stain is a crucial skill. There is no need to take more than 1 minute to do the procedure.

Ignore what you have been taught before; the following technique is as good as any for making a Gram's stain. By using this technique you will receive countless compliments from house officers regarding the quality of your stains.

1. Technique
   a. Air-dry the specimen after a thin smear has been made. Sputum smears are easily prepared by smearing the sputum sample between the two slides, or dipping a sterile cotton-tipped swab into the sputum and rubbing that across the slide
   b. *About heat fixing:* Heat fixing can introduce a lot of artifacts. If you have plenty of the specimen (e.g., urine or sputum), try it first without heat fixing and you will rarely wash off the specimen. If it is a specimen that is limited in quantity and difficult to replace (e.g., CSF), you had better heat fix so as not to incur the wrath of the house officer after you wash a valuable specimen down the sink. If an alcohol lamp is not available, you will find that alcohol pads burn wonderfully. Two to three passes through the flame are sufficient
   c. Place a liberal amount of crystal violet on the specimen; allow it to set for 10 seconds (in practice this is

usually considered the time needed to remove the cap from the next bottle)

d. Rinse with water

e. *Iodine solution:* 10 seconds

f. Rinse with water

g. Decolorize with acetone/alcohol solution, i.e., rinse until the blue color has stopped running off

h. Rinse with water

i. *Safranine:* 5 seconds

j. Rinse with water

k. Although air drying is preferable, you can carefully blot dry with a piece of filter paper if you are in a hurry

l. A good Gram's stain is characterized by PMNs that are pink with just a hint of blue in their nuclei. Remember, if the slide is less than perfect, you can simply repeat the procedure

B. PERIPHERAL BLOOD SMEAR

The ability to make a good peripheral blood smear is important. You should probably make a smear on all of your patients. This skill takes practice—don't be discouraged.

1. Technique
    a. Stick patient's finger with a lance. (*Note:* The tip of the finger hurts more, but also gives more blood.)
    b. Before making each smear, wipe the old blood from the finger with dry gauze.
    c. Use two coverslips; put a small drop of blood in the center of the first coverslip by touching it to the blood on the finger (you may need to gently squeeze the finger).
    d. Now place the second coverslip on top of the first.
    e. Let the blood spread out until it has almost stopped spreading.
    f. Now pull a corner of coverslip 1 and a corner of coverslip 2 in opposite directions. The pull is very important; the force should be parallel to the sheet of blood and

and *both* coverslips should be pulled at the same time.

g. This procedure should result in two good smears.

2. Staining
   a. Select several good smears to stain.
   b. Put the coverslips face up on corks (using corks is important to get a good dome—see discussion that follows).
   c. Apply a liberal amount of Wright's stain. It is important to create a high dome of Wright's stain on the smear. Allow it to sit 1 minute.
   d. Then add an amount of water equal to the amount of Wright's stain (keeping a high dome).
   e. Gently blow on your smears to mix the water and stain.
   f. Again add water in an amount equal to the original Wright's stain (keeping dome; you now have 2:1 or 3:1 water:Wright's).
   g. Blow gently again to mix.
   h. Now look for the formation of a shiny scum on the mixture—if you don't get a good scum, you won't get a good stain.
   i. Allow the stain to set 3 to 4 minutes after the scum appears.
   j. Rinse with water and wipe off the *back* of the coverslips with an alcohol pad if necessary.
   k. Mount smears face down, using a drop of mounting glue on a microscope slide.

3. Hints
   a. Why use a finger stick? (a) Blood from a purple top tube (which contains EDTA) will show artifacts of WBC and platelet morphology. (b) Blood with no anticoagulant, if not *very fresh*, will have platelet clumping.
   b. Make a lot of smears because only a few will turn out the way you want.
   c. The Wright's stain goes bad if not cared for properly. The top of the container must always be kept securely

closed. Use a new container when available. Bad stain will not stain the WBC nuclei adequately. You may want to keep a small bottle for yourself so that you know the lid has always been kept on tightly.

d. Clean coverslips help. Wipe your coverslips with an alcohol pad and dry them with a dry gauze pad before using them. You can do this well in advance of preparing the smear and you can keep your own supply of clean coverslips (protect them from dust).

C. BLOOD DRAWING

Blood drawing is the ultimate scut, but you must master this task. Remember one of the criteria patients use to judge their physicians is the level of pain inflicted. If you can draw blood relatively quickly and painlessly, your patients will be forever grateful.

Needles come in different sizes and styles. All styles are measured by their gauge—the larger the gauge, the smaller the diameter of the needle. Styles are mentioned in the following discussion.

Blood tubes are classified by the color of the rubber stopper in the tube which in turn signifies which chemicals, if any, are already in the tube. Whenever you draw blood, you must be sure that you are putting it into the proper tube. Some of the more common types of tubes used are in the following list, but hospitals vary so you need to check your lab's requirements.

- *Red (orange) stopper:* The familiar "red top tube" contains no chemicals so the blood will clot. This tube is used for measurements of serum such as electrolytes, most "chemistries," and serology measurements

- *Purple (lavender) stopper:* The anticoagulant EDTA in this tube allows it to be used for measurements of the formed blood elements such as CBC

- *Light blue stopper:* Contains calcium citrate and is used for coagulation studies (PT/PTT). Be sure to fill this tube to exactly where the vacuum pulls in the blood to get accurate results

- *Grey stopper:* Contains sodium fluoride. Sometimes used for glucose measurements
- *Yellow Stopper:* Used for blood cultures in some hospitals

---

To prevent clotting all tubes containing anticoagulants should be thoroughly mixed as soon as the blood is put into them. When filling a group of tubes from a syringe, fill those tubes containing an anticoagulant first.

Transferring blood from syringes to tubes should be done with a large-gauge needle (at least 20 gauge). Never push on the syringe; the tubes are evacuated and will suck the blood in. If you push or use a small needle, hemolysis will result. Purple- and blue-topped tubes need to be filled with the maximum amount of blood that they will pull in. Red-topped tubes can have less.

Blood can be drawn using one of three needle types: a standard needle with a syringe, a butterfly needle with a syringe, and a Vacutainer. Regardless of the type of needle used, several principles are followed. First find a vein. This may seem obvious, but failure at this step is the most common problem in drawing blood. Apply a tourniquet proximal to the area where you want to draw blood.

Then carefully locate potential veins. If no veins are readily apparent by inspection or palpation, gently slapping the skin where you suspect veins may be will often make them stand up. Before moving on to more drastic measures, don't forget to look at the other arm. Keeping the arms in a dependent position helps. Sometimes wrapping the arm in a warm towel to cause the veins to dilate is necessary. If no superficial veins can be found on the arms, a femoral stick can be performed (clear this with the house officer first). The femoral vein is located just medial to the femoral artery and can be carefully aspirated.

For routine venipuncture, prepping the site with an alcohol

swab is sufficient. For blood cultures and IVs, Betadine should be used.

A *butterfly needle* consists of a needle, plastic wings, and a length of plastic tubing. Using a butterfly and a syringe to draw blood is a good technique for beginners and for patients with small veins (e.g., in pediatrics).

1. Technique
   a. Connect the butterfly to a syringe.
   b. Grasp the wings with your thumb and forefinger, holding them together with the bevel up.
   c. Puncture the skin over a vein. This is the most painful part of the procedure, so the puncture should be quick and authoritative.
   d. Your angle of entry should be about 30° to the skin. Push the needle forward until it enters the vein. You will know you are in the vein because blood will immediately enter the tubing.
   e. The blood may now be gently sucked into the syringe.
   f. Should you miss the vein, pull the needle back until the tip is just beneath the skin (don't pull the needle all the way out). Relocate the vein and try again.

When using a regular *needle and syringe* basically follow the same technique as the butterfly and syringe. One slight disadvantage is that you must apply gentle suction to the syringe in order to get a blood return (and to know that you are in the vein).

The *Vacutainer* technique is generally used once you have mastered the basics of blood drawing. This apparatus consists of a plastic cylinder, a double-pointed needle, and the collecting tube. First, put the apparatus together, with the tube inside the cylinder. Push the needle through the skin (and into the vein when you become more experienced). Then push the tube forward in the cylinder so that the rubber stopper is punctured by the other point of the needle. If you are in the vein the tube will fill with blood. If not, maneuver the main needle until you enter the vein. Once the tube's stopper is punctured be careful not to pull the needle out of the skin because the vacuum in the tube will be lost. You may draw many tubes of blood with one stick by simply changing tubes.

D. STARTING IVS

Intravenous procedures can be difficult for the novice scutboy. If you are patient and know exactly where the vein you are going for is located, you should do well. There are two basic types of IV apparatus: butterflies and angiocaths.

Whichever technique you use, you should collect everything you need beforehand. You will need the needle (have two or three handy), tourniquets, bag of IV fluid, extension tubing, stopcock, IV tubing, tape of various sizes, Betadine, several 4 x 4 gauze pads, a 2 x 2 gauze pad, and a "Chux" (paper diaper, to keep blood from getting on the bed). First, set everything up and run the tubing through with fluid (eliminating bubbles). Next rip off several pieces of tape and stick them to your clothing so that they will be handy when you need them.

The *butterfly IV* procedure is quite similar to drawing blood with a butterfly. Just tape the butterfly in place once it is in the vein. Butterflies are generally easier to place than angiocaths but don't last as long because they tend to fall out of the vein.

When using an *angiocath,* first locate a good vein after applying a tourniquet. The "intern's vein" on the radial side of the wrist is always popular and therefore is often the first to be used up. Before giving up on the arm, look at the volar forearm out near the ulnar edge. Next look for good hand veins or upper arm veins. Use of the leg and foot veins is discouraged. Save the antecubital veins for blood drawing.

1. Angiocath Technique
   a. Cleanse the site with Betadine.
   b. Anesthetize the site of entry with intradermal lidocaine using a tuberculin syringe. This step is often skipped, but makes the procedure much more pleasant for the patient.

   c. Select the proper size of angio. An 18 gauge is needed for blood transfusions; a 20 gauge is usually satisfactory for other uses.

   d. Open the angiocath; separate catheter from needle to be sure that they will slide apart when necessary and then carefully place the needle back in the catheter.

When starting an angiocath (or an intracath—often used for central lines), never pull the catheter back over the needle. Its tip can be sheared off creating an embolus.

---

   e. Put the angio first through the skin above the vein. Then enter the vein. The easiest spot is in the crotch where two veins join to make one. Once the vein is entered you will get a blood return. Advance the needle very slightly (1 to 2 mm); then advance the catheter without moving the needle, i.e., slide the catheter forward off the needle—*never retreat*. (It should slide easily.) Connect the tubing and start fluid running.

   f. Be sure that the line functions properly by opening it all the way and seeing that it flows easily without causing swelling or discomfort around the IV site. Then drop the IV bag below the level of the IV briefly and see that a prompt blood return occurs assuring good placement of the catheter in the vein.

   g. Tape the catheter in place.
      (1) Use a ¼ x 3-inch piece of tape—face up under the catheter, around wings and forward. This step is critical, since the piece of tape anchors the catheter in place.
      (2) Use a 2 x 2 gauze pad with Betadine ointment to cover skin at the entry site; tape down.
      (3) Curve tubing back and tape down.
      (4) Use 4 x 4 gauze pad to cover all.
      (5) Tape 4 x 4 with several pieces of tape.

The *heparin lock* or "heplock" consists of an IV modified so that repeated injections can be made through the catheter without the need for continuous flowing IV fluid. A short piece of tubing with an injection site is kept filled with a dilute heparin solution, thus any intravenous medications can be given easily. Unless your patient needs IV fluid, this is the best way to give most IV medications. A heplock can also be used to draw repeated blood samples, such as for a glucose tolerance test (GTT).

E. IV FLUIDS

IV fluids have a nomenclature that is actually quite simple once it is understood. All solutions are identified by a combination of letters and numbers.

Examples are: *D5 W:* 5 percent dextrose in water; this solution is isotonic but the dextrose is metabolized, so this is like giving free water

NS or 0.9 percent saline → isotonic ("normal") saline solution 9 g/L = 155 mEq/L Na

D5 ½ NS is the same as *D5 0.45 NS*

D5 ¼ NS is the same as *D5 0.2 NS*

The above are the most common standard solutions. Other components may be added (e.g., KCl, specified in mEq/L). Lactated Ringer's solution simulates normal electrolyte concentrations and is often used for surgical patients.

F. FEVER WORK-UP

"I'll call the doctor in the morning. I've got a fever." — Flaming Groovies — "Slow Death."

One of the great thorns in the side of the scutboy is the night-time fever. This fever must be evaluated quickly and efficiently. A complete fever work-up follows, which may be modified according to the patient.

1. *Talk to the patient:* Ask about any pain, shortness of breath, cough, urinary tract symptoms, painful IV sites

2. Look over the recent orders in the patient's chart and the drug list. Drug fevers are commonly overlooked

---

Fevers may not be serious. Atelectasis or an inflamed IV site might be the simple cause.

---

3. *Physical exam:* Concentrate on the lungs (atelectasis or pneumonia or both), skin (e.g., decubitus lesions), recent surgical or other wounds, and the abdomen. Carefully inspect all IV sites. Naturally the patient should be assessed as to the degree of illness. Don't forget to check for meningeal signs

4. Blood cultures and perhaps a WBC with differential (see discussion, p. 89)

5. *Look at the urine:* UTIs are a common source of fever in hospitalized patients and should be taken seriously since they can lead to sepsis. Send a urine specimen to be cultured even if the urine appears to be normal and no other source is found

6. *Look at the sputum:* If the sputum looks at all questionable (e.g., PMNs), send a specimen for culture

7. In the event of a questionable chest exam, sputum, or any suspicion of pneumonia or aspiration, get a CXR

8. If the search does not produce a likely source for the fever you may elect not to treat the patient further. If you find a

likely source or if the patient appears quite ill, you will probably elect to begin treatment (the nature of which is beyond the scope of this manual). Remember, all cultures should be collected before any antibiotics are given.

G. BLOOD CULTURES

Blood cultures are the bane of medical students and house staff because they usually have to be done around 3 A.M. The secret to making this task less painful for yourself is to *be prepared.* Get a box and put all the material you will need into the box (see the discussion of the scutbox, p. 91).

Blood to be cultured is drawn sterilely, after you carefully sterilize the skin around the penetration site.

When do you draw a blood culture? Blood cultures are the intern's security blanket. If a patient spikes a fever in the middle of the night and the intern cannot think of anything else to do, he or she will draw cultures to absolve his or her conscience and look good on rounds the next morning. Blood cultures should be drawn on any *new* fevers (fever defined as 38C or 100.4F). If a patient spikes a fever every night, some clinical judgment is required. If the peak temperature is decreasing, or if you seriously doubt infection as a cause of the fever, you can stop culturing. Any change in the fever curve requires new cultures. In old people who can't mount a fever response, clinical judgment is required.

Usually two or four "sets" of cultures are drawn on admission if an infection is suspected. Subsequent cultures are done in sets of two. One "set" includes one anaerobic and one aerobic culture.

Different hospitals have different definitions of what comprises a "set." Some hospitals have cultures collected in only one tube and the lab distributes the contents to the different media. In any case, you should always do blood cultures in pairs, so that positive cultures can be interpreted more easily.

To draw blood cultures, first find a table and a trash can. Then find an area on the patient's arm that has one or preferably two good veins. The rest of the procedure is outlined as follows:

1. Technique
   a. Sterilely open several 4 x 4 gauze pad packages and lay them on the table. Pour out a generous amount of Betadine on the pads. Pick up a pad by the four corners and clean off the top of *one* of the culture bottles. Do this for each bottle, using a new pad for each. Some hospitals have prepackaged Betadine swabs (God bless them!).
   b. Set up your needle and syringe. If you are going to draw cultures one by one, you can use regular needles. If you want to draw them two at a time, use butterflies.
   c. Have several extra 20-gauge needles available.
   d. Apply a tourniquet and locate the veins.
   e. Using fresh Betadine-soaked gauze pads, clean off the skin over and around the vein (try to sterilize at least a 10-square cm area). The proper way to sterilize is to place the gauze at the center of the field and clean in gradually larger spirals. The skin should be cleaned with Betadine three times, swabbed once with alcohol, and allowed to dry.
   f. Take one of the needle/syringe set-ups and *without touching the patient's skin* insert the needle. Once the needle is in the skin, you can carefully touch the skin to locate the vein. *Don't touch the needle.*
   g. Draw 10 cc of blood. If you are using a regular needle, release the tourniquet and withdraw the needle.
   h. Now change needles and using a fresh needle put the blood into the culture tube. A Vacutainer may be used if you prefer—but do only one blood culture per venipuncture. The Vacutainer technique is best if you need to get additional bloods, but always get the culture first.
   i. *Some more hints:* Don't draw 20 cc of blood and use it for two sets of cultures. If you have a contaminant, it may grow in all bottles and confuse the picture. If you only have a few ccs of blood because you blew a vein,

use it anyway. Even the best of us get a contaminant into a culture at some time or other (usually staphylococcus epidermidis, streptococcus, or diphtheroids). Don't worry too much about it, but try to be more careful next time.

H. THE SCUTBOX

A box, known as the scutbox because it contains the items you will commonly use at the hospital, is a real time-saver. At 3 A.M. you don't feel like chasing down everything needed for doing blood cultures or starting IVs. The layout pictured on page 92 is suggested by Dr. Paul Scanlon.

Note: The box does not contain a bottle for used needles, although this can be included. Always remove used needles with the Halsted clamp—*never* with your fingers. (Who was Halsted???)

I. ARTERIAL BLOOD GASES

The keys to doing a blood gas quickly are to precisely locate the artery and to have a steady hand. As usual, you must have all your equipment ready before you start. You will need a cup of ice and a blood gas kit.

To obtain an arterial sample for an ABG you need a heparinized syringe. A glass syringe is desirable if it is available; a glass syringe will passively fill with arterial blood (thus assuring you that you are in the artery). Whether using a glass or a plastic syringe, first put about 1 cc of 1:1000 heparin into the syringe. Now remove most of the heparin and any air bubbles present. Next attach the needle you wish to use. A standard 22-gauge needle can be used with a glass syringe. However, a 23-gauge butterfly (with the tubing half filled with heparin) is preferable with a plastic syringe, because the arterial blood will pulsate in the butterfly tubing, thus assuring you that you are in the artery.

Now, select the artery you wish to use. Unless this is a cardiac

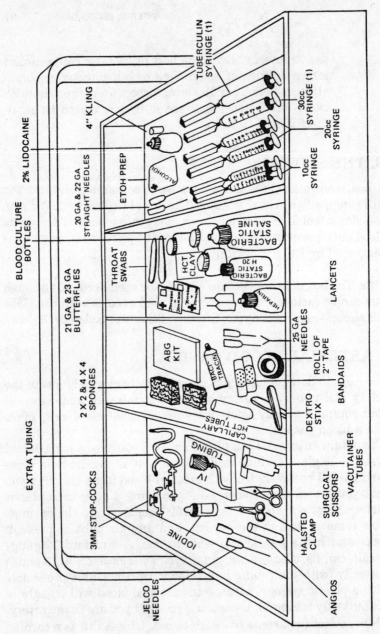

TUBERCULIN SYRINGE (1)

30cc SYRINGE (1)

20cc SYRINGE

10cc SYRINGE

2% LIDOCAINE

4" KLING

ETOH PREP

ALCOHOL

20 GA & 22 GA STRAIGHT NEEDLES

BLOOD CULTURE BOTTLES

THROAT SWABS

BACTERIOSTATIC SALINE

HCT CLAY H20

BACTERIOSTATIC H20

HEPARIN

21 GA & 23 GA BUTTERFLIES

LANCETS

25 GA NEEDLES

ABG KIT

BACITRACIN

ROLL OF 2" TAPE

BANDAIDS

2 X 2 & 4 X 4 SPONGES

DEXTRO STIX

CAPILLARY HCT TUBES

VACUTAINER TUBES

EXTRA TUBING

IV TUBING

SURGICAL SCISSORS

HALSTED CLAMP

3MM STOP-COCKS

IODINE

ANGIOS

JELCO NEEDLES

92

arrest case, don't use the femoral artery. You can use either the brachial or radial artery. The advantage of the radial artery is that if trauma causes spasm or a clot, blood will still be supplied to the hand via the ulnar artery. If the brachial artery clots off, however, you may have big trouble. (The advantage of the brachial artery is that it is bigger and much easier to hit.)

If you use the radial artery, have the patient supinate the arm and extend the wrist by resting it on something (traditionally a roll of toilet paper). Carefully locate the artery and maintain control of it by keeping it between your index and middle fingers. The spot where the artery is closest to the surface is usually 1 to 2 cm proximal to the wrist. When you've located the artery, clean off the area quickly with the Betadine and then with an alcohol swab. Then pull up a chair and *sit down.* Again, control the artery by keeping it between your fingers. Hold the syringe like a pencil in your other hand. Hold the needle directly over the artery at about the same angle as a pencil, with the point directed *against* the flow of blood. Quickly push the needle through the skin *only.* Then, using one finger, again locate the artery and slowly advance the needle. When you hit the artery, blood will pulse into the syringe; this pulse, along with the brighter red color of the blood, is how you can tell that you have hit the artery rather than a vein. If you get no return after inserting the needle past where the artery should be, relocate the artery and decide which side of the needle it is on. Then pull the needle back to the skin (but not out) and again slowly advance the needle. Never aspirate with a glass syringe while obtaining an ABG. If you are in an artery, the arterial pressure will fill the syringe without your help. You must pull on a plastic syringe (because of its increased resistance) so other methods (e.g., pulsation in butterfly tubing) must be used to be sure of arterial—not venous—puncture. You need about 2 cc of blood.

When measuring gases, always wait at least 20 minutes after changing the oxygen content of inspired air before checking blood gas. If you have a small air bubble in the syringe after drawing the arterial blood, stick the needle through an alcohol swab. Point the syringe upward and carefully eject the bubble. The swab prevents blood from dribbling down the syringe onto your hands.

After you have obtained the needed blood, firmly hold a gauze pad over the artery at the site of insertion. Then remove the needle and compress the artery. The trick now is to quickly get any air out of the syringe, cap it, and put it in ice without allowing a huge hematoma to form at the arterial site. This can be done in a few different ways: (1) Have a nurse hold the gauze; (2) Have the patient hold it (usually not very satisfactory); (3) You hold it; one trick is to lean your elbow on the artery, thus freeing both hands. It is recommended that the artery be held for 5 minutes. Place the syringe in ice as soon as possible.

J. NASOGASTRIC TUBE

Inserting a nasogastric (NG) tube is one of the most unpleasant tasks for both the patient and the scutboy. Often, merely the threat of an NG tube will make mysterious abdominal pain "magically" vanish. The procedure is as follows:

1. *You will need:* Disposable gloves, two emesis basins (one filled with ice and one available for the patient to use, if needed), a 50-cc syringe, Xylocaine spray, lubricant, and an NG tube.

2. Place the distal end of the tube in the ice-filled basin. This step will freeze a gentle curve in the tube and allow it to follow the curve of the nasopharynx.

3. While waiting for the tube to freeze have the patient sit facing you and spray the Xylocaine into the nasopharynx.

4. Remove the tube from the ice and squirt lubricant on it.

5. PUT ON YOUR GLOVES!

6. Ease the NG tube into the nose and gradually push the

tube in. Push the tube in a medial plane, i.e., along the nasal septum. You may encounter some resistance, but *don't force* the tube (there have been cases where the cribriform plexus was pierced).

7. When the tube moves to the epiglottis, ask the patient to take a big swallow. Quickly push the tube down the esophagus into the stomach. To determine that it is in the right place, inject 50 cc of air while listening over the stomach. If the tube is in the stomach you will hear bubbling.

8. Clamp the tube (unless it is to be connected to suction) and tape it to the nose.

9. If the tube isn't in the stomach it may be in one of three places:
   a. *The lung:* The patient will be coughing vigorously. Pull back and try again. One suggestion is to have the patient lean his or her head further forward.
   b. *The mouth:* Try again.
   c. *The brain:* Call the resident.

K. ARTERIAL LINE

This is an advanced scutboy technique. Before attempting this, you must master blood gases and IVs.

Arterial lines are glorified IVs that are placed in arteries instead of veins. They are used almost exclusively with patients in the intensive care setting. Usually these patients require constant BP monitoring or frequent blood gases.

Ask the nurse on duty to collect all the necessary equipment and to have everything ready for the catheter insertion *before you begin.* This includes a pressure gauge, monitor equipment, tubing, and tape. You should use an 18- or 20-gauge arterial catheter.

1. The radial artery is the most common site for an arterial line. However, you must be sure that the patient has an

intact ulnar artery before attempting the procedure. Radial artery spasm is a common complication (more so than with blood gases) and could be disastrous.

2. The radial artery should be located as with a blood gas, prepped with Betadine, and sterilely draped. Put on sterile gloves and anesthetize the skin over the artery with lidocaine.

3. Insert the catheter through the anesthetized skin directly over the artery. The catheter should be held at an angle of about 30° and directed *against* the flow of blood. When you get blood return, flatten the angle until the needle is nearly parallel to the skin and advance about 1 mm. The Teflon catheter can then be advanced (like an IV) into the artery. Actually, this is a little trickier than advancing an IV and is usually the place where novice scutboys run into trouble.

4. Once the catheter is in the artery, immediately connect the tubing to the line. If this is not done quickly, you will learn approximately how long it takes a person to exsanguinate.

5. Anchor the line with sutures. Cover with a sterile gauze pad and tape down.

L. LUMBAR PUNCTURE

1. Most hospitals have LP trays that contain everything you need to do a lumbar puncture: tubes, spinal needle, manometer, lidocaine, 22- and 25-gauge needles, syringe, 3-way stopcock.

2. Before attempting an LP, be sure that the patient's clotting parameters are adequate (platelets >50,000 and PT <15 seconds). Subdural hematomas can be disastrous, so transfuse with platelets or fresh frozen plasma if needed. Also, people with suspected mass lesions, papilledema, or focal neurologic findings should have a CT scan before you attempt an LP.

3. Proper positioning of the patient is vital. The patient should lie on his or her side, curled up in the fetal position. Often a nurse is needed to maximally flex the patient's head. Violent patients may require two or three people to hold them.

4. One handy tip is to tell patients that the procedure is very safe, AS LONG AS THEY STAY PERFECTLY STILL! You will be amazed how quickly that will quiet an agitated patient.

5. The spinal cord extends to about L-1 or L-2 in most people. Therefore the L3-4 and L4-5 interspaces are usually safe for your procedure. L-5 usually lies on a line that connects the patient's iliac crests.

6. Make an indentation into the skin just above the spinous process of L-5 with an unopened pen. If the interspace seems small or calcified, try one interspace higher. The most common problem encountered is total obscuration of landmarks by obesity. In this case, locate the midline and make a mark where you guess L-5 should be!

7. Prep a generous area with Betadine.

8. Anesthetize the skin with lidocaine using a 22-gauge needle, then anesthetize the deeper ligaments. These are fairly insensitive to pain, and little anesthesia is needed beyond the skin.

9. Using a 20- or 22-gauge spinal needle, pierce the skin just rostral to the spinous process. The bevel should be up so that the fibers of the dura are separated rather than sheared.

10. Control the needle by holding the point of insertion between your two index fingers and the hub of the needle between your thumbs. This gives exquisite control even to those with significant tremors.

11. Angle the needle so that the point is inclined cephalad about 30° off center. If you use L4-5, it is about equivalent to aiming for the umbilicus. You *must* stay in the longitudinal plane of the spine.

12. Quickly advance the needle between 1 and 2 cm. Withdraw the stylet and look for CSF return. If nothing returns, replace the stylet and advance 1 or 2 mm and repeat this ritual.

13. Eventually you will hit:
    a. *A nerve:* The patient will scream in agony about pain radiating down one leg. This means that the needle is out of the longitudinal plane. If the right leg hurts withdraw the needle to just beneath the skin and direct it more toward the patient's left (or vice versa).
    b. *Bone:* This is the most common difficulty. Either pull out and try a steeper angle or try to march over the bone. Occasionally you may have to use a different interspace, if ligaments are heavily calcified. If you continuously hit bone, sit the patient up and repeat the same procedure. Many LPs that are difficult to do with the patient lying down are easy with the patient sitting. Don't bother checking opening pressure if the patient is sitting.
    c. *Pulsatile blood:* Oops! Withdraw the needle, send a tube of venous blood to the blood bank for T&C and pray.
    d. *Nothing:* Can happen if the patient is massively obese. A longer needle can be used.
    e. *CSF:* This is usually clear liquid that slowly drips from the needle. You often feel a pop as the needle pierces the dura.

A correctly placed needle never needs to be forced.

---

14. Check the opening pressure with the manometer. This can

take a minute or so to equilibrate and should have respiratory variation. If the pressure is very high (i.e., approaching 300 mm) remove as little fluid as necessary, check a closing pressure, and get help. Rapid pressure changes can lead to herniation and death, so it is a good idea to notify your resident before collecting fluid if the opening pressure is high.

15. If the pressure is normal, remove the manometer (it's OK to spill the CSF as long as the patient doesn't have Jakob-Creutzfeldt disease). Collect the fluid as described in "Fluid Work-Up," p. 107. If the first tube is blood-tinged or if you in any way suspect a traumatic tap, be sure to send the first and last tubes for cell counts.

16. If the fluid stops dripping, you can have the patient take a few deep breaths or gently rotate the needle.

17. When completed, reinsert the stylet and remove the needle.

18. Place an adhesive bandage over the site and have the patient lie flat for about 6 hours. Post-LP headaches are usually due to CSF leak after the needle is removed, and begin about a day later. Between 30 and 50 cc of CSF leaks even under optimum conditions. The higher gauge (22-gauge) needles have a lower incidence of complications. However, they are more flexible and more difficult to control.

19. Occasionally everybody will have difficulty. If you miss after two or three passes, get help from the intern or resident. They may attempt the LP with the patient in the sitting position (as for a thoracentesis) or via the lateral approach.

20. If performed properly, the LP is a remarkable safe procedure. Remember, though, that any break in sterility can lead to serious bacterial meningitis. All LPs should be supervised by a house officer.

M. THORACENTESIS

1. This procedure is performed in order to remove pleural fluid for either diagnostic (to examine the fluid) or therapeutic reasons (to remove fluid that is compromising the patient's respiratory status).

2. Complications are common even in experienced hands.

3. Get decubitus x-rays (views with the patient lying on his or her side) to be sure that the fluid "layers out"—i.e., is free flowing. If the effusion is loculated, ultrasound can be used to locate the pocket precisely.

4. As with all invasive procedures be sure that the patient has normal coagulation studies and platelet count.

5. To begin the procedure, have the patient sit on the edge of the bed with feet dangling and body leaning forward onto a pillow on a table.

6. Percuss the effusion and locate its upper border. You should enter at the posterior axillary line into the first or second interspace below the superior border of the dullness to percussion. If you go too high your risk of pneumothorax is increased; if you go too low you could hit the liver or spleen. Try to avoid inserting the needle below the 8th interspace.

7. Prep and drape the patient. This is a sterile procedure.

8. Infiltrate the skin with lidocaine. Then insert a small needle (22-gauge) and infiltrate lidocaine into the periosteum of the rib below the interspace. March up and over the rib, infiltrating with lidocaine and aspirating as you advance. When you get free flow of fluid, you have then precisely located the effusion and are in the pleural space. If air returns, withdraw the needle and obtain a chest x-ray to evaluate for a probable pneumothorax. Occasionally a pa-

tient will be too fat for the 1½" needles and no fluid will be obtained. A spinal needle can be used *carefully* in its place. Remember to go *over the rib, not under* it, or you might hit an intercostal artery or nerve.

9. Once you have located the fluid, there are three basic techniques for obtaining an adequate specimen; the same principles as those used to locate fluid should be used in each technique.

   a. *Metal needle:* This is best used for diagnostic taps in which small amounts of fluid are quickly obtained (the "in and out" tap). Go over the rib and slowly insert the needle as you gently aspirate with the syringe. As soon as you get fluid into the syringe, stop advancing. You can put a Kelly clamp on the needle at skin level so you cannot accidentally push the needle in further and hit the lung. Withdraw the fluid needed for your diagnostic tests (usually should include pH).

Patients with asymptomatic effusion may develop inspiratory pain after thoracentesis because of contact between the pleura.

---

   b. *Angiocath:* This technique allows you to safely remove larger amounts of fluid. Insert the angiocath, with a syringe attached to the needle, as described previously. When fluid is obtained, remove the stylet and attach a syringe to the catheter. The patient should be instructed to hold his or her breath during this step, and you should put a finger over the catheter. If the patient takes a deep breath at this point a pneumothorax could result. With the plastic catheter your chances of puncturing the lung are much less.

   c. *Intercath:* This is a long catheter that can be threaded through the needle into the pleural space. Many hospitals have special kits that contain everything you need.

Insert the large-bore needle into the pleural space as previously described and advance the catheter. Once the catheter is in the space, the needle is withdrawn and a needle guard is placed on it to prevent shearing off the catheter. The other end of the catheter can then be connected to a vacuum bottle via extension tubing and the effusion "tapped dry."

10. The pleural fluid should be examined as described in "Fluid Work-Up," p. 107. You should order the studies that are relevant for your patient, instead of having a "blanket" fluid work-up. Save some fluid; other people (such as residents and attendings) may define relevant differently than you do.

11. Always get a CXR after any thoracentesis or attempt. A small pneumothorax will probably require no treatment but a large one will warrant insertion of a chest tube.

N. PARACENTESIS

There are a variety of clinical situations in which paracentesis is necessary. We will describe a few of the many approaches to obtaining peritoneal fluid.

1. *Is there ascites?* Often there is little question as to the presence of ascites on physical exam. In subtler cases, there are several noninvasive techniques. A flat plate of the abdomen is the simplest and easiest to obtain, but also the least sensitive. Signs such as obscuration of the psoas muscle margin are clues for the experienced observer. U/S can locate and identify free fluid. If in doubt, a paracentesis can be performed with a small needle to see if fluid is present.

2. Preparing the patient
   a. Before attempting paracentesis, you must check clotting parameters. The most common complication is *bleeding*, not perforated bowel. If the PT is prolonged,

fresh frozen plasma should be given to bring it at least to within 1½ to 2 times control. If the platelet count is low secondary to hypersplenism, platelet transfusions will be of little benefit.

b. Have the patient empty his or her bladder (by straight cath if necessary). This is particularly important if the midline approach is used.

c. Position the patient so that the location of the tap is as dependent as possible. This is not terribly important in patients with massive ascites. Even so, if the midline approach is used, the patient should be supine and propped up in bed to about 45°. This brings the fluid to the dependent portion of the abdomen and allows bowel loops to float harmlessly away. If the lateral approach is used, the patient should be positioned in the left lateral decubitus position, while sitting up as in the midline approach. The dependent portion of the abdomen, usually the left lower quadrant, can then be tapped.

d. Percuss the area you wish to tap. If it is resonant, you run the risk of aspirating bowel content. Reposition the patient.

3. Midline approach

a. Position the patient for the midline approach.

b. Prepare a generous area from above the umbilicus to the symphysis pubis with Betadine.

c. Anesthesize a small area of skin (two thirds the distance *from* the symphysis pubis to the umbilicus with lidocaine. Avoid surgical scars because of possible bowel adhesions to the abdominal wall.

d. Using a 22-gauge needle and a small syringe filled with lidocaine, enter the skin at a 30° angle.

e. Track the needle rostrally subdermally for about ½ to 1 cm, then dive into the abdomen, perpendicular to the skin. This produces a Z-track and prevents peritoneal fluid under high pressure from leaking after the procedure.

f. Gently advance the needle, aspirating and injecting lidocaine as you go.

g. You may feel a slight pop when you enter the peritoneum. Fluid should then flow back freely into the syringe.

h. If no fluid is obtained, there are several options:
   (1) Reposition the patient.
   (2) Use a longer needle.
   (3) Try the lateral approach.
   (4) Use sonographic guidance.

i. If you hit blood, pull back immediately and try another location.

j. Once you locate fluid, withdraw the needle. If a diagnostic paracentesis is performed, use the same technique with an 18- or 20-gauge needle and a large syringe.

k. Occasionally therapeutic paracenteses are performed to relieve tense ascites. For this you need an 18-gauge angiocath, extension tubing, and a vacuum bottle. Locate the fluid as just described, attach the angiocath to a syringe, and insert it into the abdomen. When fluid is aspirated advance the Teflon catheter and withdraw the metal stylet. Attach one end of the extension tubing to the angiocath and the other to the vacuum bottle. No more than 1 L of ascites should be removed per day.

4. Lateral approach
   a. Position the patient as previously noted for the lateral approach.
   b. Enter the abdomen one third the distance *from* the dependent anterior superior iliac spine to the umbilicus. Then Z-track rostrally or laterally to avoid the hypogastric vessels. When fluid is located, continue as with the midline approach.

5. *Dressing:* Usually an adhesive bandage will suffice. A pressure bandage should be used on patients with tense ascites.

O. ARTHROCENTESIS

Arthrocentesis consists of aspirating fluid from a joint with a needle. This procedure is generally done to help determine which type of arthritis a patient has. In many cases of chronic arthritis this procedure is not required and a diagnosis can be made by other means. However, whenever an infected (septic) joint is suspected, arthrocentesis is mandatory. Other conditions, such as gout, are best diagnosed by synovial fluid examination. All peripheral joints can be aspirated, although most physicians develop competence with only a few. The knee is the most common joint to be aspirated by those not trained in rheumatology or orthopedics, so we will use that as an example.

1. The knee is usually an easy joint to aspirate. The first step is to find the best location to insert the needle. The medial approach is commonly used. The point of needle insertion is about one third of the distance from the proximal border of the patella toward the distal border and about 1 cm deep to the medial border of the patella. This location should be marked, e.g., use a ball-point pen with the point retracted. During the procedure the patient is supine with the knee fully extended and relaxed.

2. Arthrocentesis should be considered a sterile procedure. The area should be cleaned carefully with Betadine. Sterile gloves are advisable to reinforce the concept of sterility.

3. The skin surface should be anesthetized with either ethyl chloride spray or a bleb of lidocaine.

4. A 19 to 22 gauge needle is attached to a syringe of a size that should be able to hold the amount of fluid that appears to be in the joint (10 to 60 cc).

5. Insert the needle into the area you marked and push stead-

ily forward while applying gentle suction with the syringe. When the joint space is entered, synovial fluid will flow easily into the syringe.

6. In general you should remove as much fluid as possible. This may require minor adjustment in the position of the needle.

7. After the fluid appears to have been fully aspirated, remove the needle and apply an adhesive bandage.

8. Analysis of the synovial fluid is the whole purpose of the procedure, so do it carefully. The appearance of the fluid is one of the most critical observations. Normal fluid is yellow and clear. Abnormal synovial fluid is classified as group I (noninflammatory), group II (inflammatory), and group III (purulent). As the fluid becomes more inflammatory it becomes cloudier and less viscous. Hemorrhagic fluid (sometimes referred to as group IV) usually indicates trauma or a "traumatic tap." Some conditions may produce synovial fluid with an unusual appearance (e.g., brown synovial fluid in villonodular synovitis). In any case, carefully noting the appearance of the fluid and its volume is essential.

9. The most important routine lab test is the synovial fluid cell count which often allows for separation of the fluid into one of the three aforementioned categories. Frequently, fluid is sent for such studies as glucose and protein levels, but the value of these determinations is not always clear.

10. If infection is being considered, a portion of the fluid should be sent for cultures and a Gram's stain carefully examined.

11. Examination of the fluid for crystals should be routine since crystal-induced disease (especially gout) can mimic everything from rheumatoid arthritis to septic joints. Unfortunately, crystal examination is done poorly by many hospital labs.

This is an examination technique you should master.

Often the hardest part is locating a polarizing microscope. A drop of fluid is placed on a microscope slide that has been wiped off with a piece of lens paper (dirt may look like crystals). A clean coverslip is applied. If the microscope is set up properly the background color of the entire field is red. Crystals are searched for under high power. They are small—remember they fit inside leukocytes. You are looking for intracellular crystals. Urate (gout) crystals are needle-shaped and yellow when parallel to the plane of polarization and blue when perpendicular (negatively birefringent), CPPD (pseudogout) crystals are rhomboid in shape and have the opposite color relationship to the plane of polarization.

12. Joints are often injected with steroid/lidocaine mixtures using a similar technique. Joint injections should be carried out only after consideration of the indications and possible risks in each clinical situation.

P. FLUID WORK-UP

The fluid work-up is an important scutboy duty. Fluids can come from the pleural space, peritoneal cavity, CSF, joints, etc. Each type of fluid has a different work-up; however all fluids need a basic work-up done by you. In addition to sending fluid samples for various lab studies (culture, cytology, chemistry, etc.), you should perform the following.

1. *Cell count:* For this you need a microscope, counting chamber (hemacytometer), stain (Turk's solution) and a few pipettes. Clean and dry the counting chamber and place the coverslip on it. Draw a couple of drops of fluid into a pipette and touch the pipette to part A (see diagram, p. 108).

   Capillary action will draw the fluid into that half of the chamber. Now look at this part of the counting chamber with the microscope. If there are no cells, your cell count is zero (normal for CSF) and you are finished. If cells are

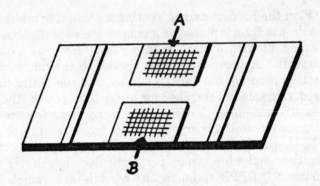

present, count the red cells and white cells (although you may have trouble differentiating mononuclear from polymorphonuclear cells). The cell count, in cells per cubic millimeter, is the total number of cells in the grid of the counting chamber multiplied by 10/9. If there are too many cells present to count them all, count only part of the grid and multiply appropriately. If cells are present you need to look at a stained sample. The stain will serve to lyse red cells and stain the nuclei of the white cells. Thus the stained sample allows you to make a differential WBC count and check your total WBC count from the unstained specimen. You cannot use the stained sample to count RBC (remember that the stain lysed them). To stain the fluid draw some stain into a fresh pipette and then drain the stain out, leaving the inside of the pipette coated with stain. Now draw up the fluid to be counted into the pipette and sufficient stain should remain to stain the fluid. Many hospital labs centrifuge CSF and Wright's stain a sample to obtain a highly accurate differential.

2. *Gram's stain:* See discussion beginning on p. 79.

3. *India ink—for CSF:* The india ink test is a simple method to look for *Cryptococcus* (which is a common etiologic agent of meningitis in many teaching hospitals). Place a couple of

drops of CSF on a slide, mix it with a drop of india ink, and cover with a coverslip. Examine the slide under low and high power. *Cryptococcus* is a small sphere (about the size of a WBC) surrounded by a larger clear capsule. Often, unspun specimens are negative, and the organism is seen only after centrifugation. Also, cryptococcal antigen can be positive even with negative india ink preps or cultures.

Q. CENTRAL VENOUS LINES

1. This section is intended to acquaint the reader with techniques used to start central venous lines. These procedures have risks and should be done with a more experienced person present until you are comfortable with the procedure.

2. A CVP (central venous pressure) line is a long catheter inserted into the superior vena cava via the internal jugular or subclavian vein.

3. Several features are shared by all approaches to the central line:
    a. *Needle and catheter:* Instead of using a standard angiocath (as used with peripheral IVs) an intracath is used. This consists of a large-gauge needle (usually a #14) *through* which the plastic catheter is introduced. The needle is removed once the catheter is in place.
    b. Use a *small* needle to explore. Because the veins you are aiming for are near vital structures (such as carotid arteries, lungs) it is best to locate the vein with a small-gauge needle (e.g., #22). Once the vein is located the small needle can be left in to serve as a guide for the large needle. You will find that hitting the carotid with a #22 needle is much less disconcerting than hitting it with a #14 needle. Many scutboys use the same needle that they are infiltrating lidocaine with to do the exploration.

     c. The patient should be placed in the Trendelenburg position (head down) to distend neck veins.

Because of the risk of air embolism, central lines should always be inserted or removed with the patient in the Trendelenburg position.

---

     d. This is a sterile procedure. A wide area should be prepped with Betadine, draped, and sterile gloves used.

     e. Once the procedure is complete, get a CXR to be sure there is no pneumothorax and to check the catheter position.

     f. Once the catheter is in place SUTURE IT IN!!! You don't want your GI bleeder with DTs to pull out your beautifully placed line.

4. Before beginning this procedure review an anatomy atlas to refresh your memory of the relationships of your landmarks, the veins, and the arteries. You will then be surprised that an internal jugular (IJ) line can be started without hitting the carotid!

5. The major approaches to the central line are
     a. Internal jugular–posterior approach
     b. Internal jugular–middle approach
     c. Internal jugular–anterior approach
     d. Subclavian

6. A few points about internal jugular versus the subclavian approach:
     a. The risk of pneumothorax is less with the jugular
     b. If you hit an artery the hematoma is visible with the jugular approach and is easily compressed
     c. The subclavian approach gives the patient more freedom to move his or her head

7. In general the right side is chosen for several reasons:
     a. Direct line to RA

b. Dome of lung is lower on right side

c. The thoracic duct is on the left side and is best not punctured

8. If you change sides you should first get a CXR to avoid a bilateral pneumothorax.

9. You should try each of the following techniques and then become proficient at the one you are most comfortable with.

a. *IJ—posterior approach:* Familiarize yourself with your patient's landmarks. You can define the sternocleido-mastoid more readily by having the patient twist his or her neck against pressure on his or her cheek. As with all procedures involving needles (and other sharp objects) you take your time and be sure you know where to put it.

   (1) The needle should be inserted at the posterior border of the SCM where the external jugular crosses the muscle (about one third of the way up the muscle).

   (2) First infiltrate the skin in this area with lidocaine. Then insert your needle and point it toward the suprasternal notch. The IJ is superficial, right below the muscle. Think of yourself as sliding the needle along the inner surface of the muscle.

   (3) As the needle is advanced, apply suction with a syringe. You will get blood back when you hit the vein. Next, follow the same path with the larger needle. Once you get blood back remove the syringe and thread the catheter through the needle. Keep a finger over the end of the needle during the transition from syringe to catheter to prevent air from being sucked in. *Never* pull the plastic catheter back through the needle; the tip can be sheared off. It is difficult to get a 3″ length of catheter out of a pulmonary artery.

   (4) Hook up your IV fluid to the catheter, clamp on

the needle guard, suture the catheter in place, and
dress it.
b. *IJ—middle approach:* This is a very simple technique.
Your landmark is the triangle formed by the two heads
of the SCM and the clavicle.
   (1) Insert your needle into the center of this triangle.
   (2) Point the needle along the sagittal plane, holding
   the needle and syringe at about a 30° angle to the
   skin. The IJ and subclavian veins join in this
   region so you should be able to hit one of them. If
   you get no blood return, aim more laterally (until
   you are aiming for the nipple).
   (3) Once in the vein proceed as previously described.
c. *IJ—anterior approach:* This approach is dangerous and
offers no advantage over the other two. It is best
avoided and will not be described.
d. Subclavian
   (1) The needle is introduced 1 cm below the junction
   of the medial and middle thirds of the clavicle.
   (2) Advance the needle parallel to the plane of the
   patient's back, medially toward the suprasternal
   notch.
   (3) If you hit the clavicle (which you probably should),
   march under it. The subclavian vein is tethered
   open by surrounding structures and should be easily entered even in the face of significant hypo-
   volemia.
   (4) Rotate the needle so that the bevel is caudal; insert the catheter (this helps move the needle in the
   right direction).
   (5) Withdraw the needle and proceed as previously
   described.
   (6) If you hit the carotid artery, apply firm pressure
   for 10 to 15 minutes.

10. When central lines are removed the tips should be cul-

tured. Catheters are a common source of infection. If your patient spikes a fever 6 hours after you removed the catheter it is good to know that the catheter tip is in the microbiology lab. If the catheter was the source, you should know it.

11. If a patient with a central line spikes a new fever, the line should be pulled and the tip cultured.

R. FOLEY CATHETER

1. Although insertion of a Foley catheter is often a nursing procedure, you may be called upon to perform this task.

2. A Foley is a catheter (developed by Frederick Foley, Johns Hopkins Medical School, class of 1918) that is inserted into the bladder to provide constant urinary drainage. A balloon at the top of the catheter is inflated once the catheter is inserted, to prevent the catheter from slipping out (although more than one intoxicated or demented patient has pulled an inflated Foley out).

3. A Foley catheter is *not* a benign instrument. Virtually everyone who has one in develops bacteriuria within a few days, and a certain percentage of patients will develop sepsis. It is important to keep this in mind, because most physicians have seen more complications from Foleys than from LPs, thoracenteses, etc. A Foley should be inserted only after careful thought.

4. For females, have the patient placed in the lithotomy position. Prep the labia and urethra with Betadine and sterilely insert a lubricated catheter into the urethra. When urine flow is established, inflate the balloon with sterile saline (usually 5 cc). Attach the Foley to a drainage bag in order to quantitate urine output. Tape the catheter to the patient's thigh. The key to easy and rapid catheterization is locating the urethra (check those anatomy texts!).

5. Cathing men can be a little trickier.
   a. Place a sterile towel under the penis.
   b. Prep the glans with Betadine.
   c. Position the penis so that it points toward the umbilicus.
   d. Sterilely insert the generously lubricated Foley through the meatus; most unsuccessful attempts are due to insufficient lubrication.
   e. If all goes well, the catheter will slip into the bladder, as with females.
   f. If the man is over 50 yo, chances are he will have some prostate hyperplasia. Gentle pressure can often overcome this obstacle, but *don't* force it. If this doesn't work, try a smaller catheter (#12 or #14 F). There are special catheters with tapered tips that can be used if you are still unsuccessful. Usually someone with more experience (like a resident or a urologist) will insert these.
   g. Occasionally the urethra is lacerated by the catheter and a false channel is produced. If you suspect this, a urologic consult should be obtained immediately.
   h. Hematuria, usually microscopic, is common after Foley insertion and need not cause alarm.
   i. If a patient with a Foley develops a fever, the urine is often the source.

S. HEMOCCULT AND FECAL LEUKOCYTES

The examination of stool has always held peculiar fascination for internists. The most commonly performed tests on stool are the methylene blue stain for fecal leukocytes and the Hemoccult for occult blood.

1. *Obtaining a specimen:* The easiest and least unpleasant method is to have the nurse save a specimen. This may however, take days. The more effective scutboys go straight to the source with a gloved hand.

2. *Hemoccult:* The test for occult blood has advanced considerably since the advent of Hemoccult testing paper. Before this, stool was tested with acetic acid, guaiac, and peroxide. This method was cumbersome and had up to 50 percent false positives and negatives. To use Hemoccult simply place a small sample of stool on the paper and add two drops of developer fluid. If occult blood is present, the paper will turn blue.

3. *Methylene blue:* This is a stain for fecal leukocytes and is incredibly easy to do. Simply smear a thin sample of stool on a glass slide and stain with a generous amount of methylene blue; rinse after about 30 seconds. Examine the specimen under the microscope when the slide is dry. Alternatively, place two or three drops of methylene blue on the smear and cover with a glass coverslip.

The most important part of examining the stained specimen is to ignore everything except the leukocytes. A positive smear will usually have sheets of polys. This is seen in inflammatory bowel disease and a variety of invasive infections. Viral enteritis, cholera, and malabsorption are examples of diseases in which fecal leukocytes are absent.

Note that a Wright's stain of stool is equally effective, but is time-consuming.

SECTION 3

Appendix I. Sample Write-up

A. STUDENT ADMISSION NOTE

This 53-year-old white married bricklayer is admitted to Dr. Ramone's service with an 8-hour history of acute arthritis of the right knee.

B. HISTORY OF PRESENT ILLNESS

This patient's medical history is notable for 10 years of alcohol abuse and hypertension treated intermittently with HCTZ. He was in his usual state of active good health until this morning when he noticed that his left knee was swollen and painful when he got out of bed. He went to work but the pain worsened so that at about 1 P.M. his co-workers brought him to the ER. He took some aspirin for the pain during the morning but did nothing else to treat the knee, and was standing or squatting virtually all morning. He states that the pain is now the worst that he has ever had. He had no symptoms leading to this acute knee pain and no warning that anything was wrong until this morning. He has no previous history of arthritis, but was diagnosed as having gout about 5 years ago while on vacation in Florida. At that time he had swelling and pain in his right great toe. He was seen at a walk-in clinic and given an unknown medicine that made him well in a few days. He says that the toe was not aspirated and no blood test or x-rays were done. He denies fever chills, trauma of any kind, cuts to the skin, history of kidney stones, any pain elsewhere, or FH of gout or arthritis. He has not had any alcohol to drink in a week. He has no history of back pain, morning stiffness, skin rashes, diarrhea, penile discharge, or eye inflammation.

Upon presentation to the ER he was noted to be febrile to 38.4C. X-ray of the knee was normal except for a large effusion. Arthrocentesis produced 60 cc of cloudy fluid with 70,000 WBC (98% PMNs). Gram's stain was negative. Crystal examination was not performed.

C. PAST MEDICAL HISTORY

1. *General health:* Excellent. Has not missed work in 3 years

2. Medical illness:
   a. + Hypertension x 10 years. Takes HCTZ sometimes but not in the past "couple of months"
   b. + Alcohol abuse. Drank "a lot" when younger (30 yo). Now about a six pack of beer on weekends. Never had DTs, seizures, tremulousness, or pancreatitis
   c. − Pneumonia, TB, VD, hepatitis, or DM

3. *Allergies:* Codeine causes nausea

4. *Hospitalizations and operations:* Appendectomy about 15 years ago, no complications

5. *Blood transfusions:* Unknown

6. *Serious injuries:* None

7. *Drugs:* Alcohol as above, never smoked

8. *Medications:* None at present

D. FAMILY HISTORY

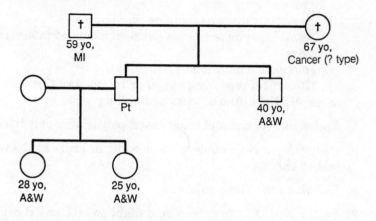

+ Ca and heart disease (see diagram)
− BP, gout, DM, asthma, or arthritis

E. SOCIAL HISTORY

1. *General:* Married x 28 years, lives with wife. HS education, Army 1953–1955 (not overseas). "Handyman" x 10 years, bricklayer since

2. *Habits:* Sleeps well. 2 to 4 cups of coffee per day

3. *Travel:* None out of US, not out of state in 3 years

F. REVIEW OF SYSTEMS

1. *Skin:* No rashes, pruritis, or alopecia

2. *Skeletal:* None except HPI

3. Head
   a. *General:* No HA, syncope, dizziness, or head injuries
   b. *Eyes:* Trouble reading close up x several years ("guess I need glasses")

    c. *Ears:* No decreased hearing, tinnitus, discharge, or vertigo

    d. *Nose:* No sinus problems, or discharge

    e. *Teeth:* No symptoms; has not seen a dentist in several years

    f. *Tongue:* No swelling or pain

    g. *Throat:* No pain, dysphagia, or recent sore throats

    h. *Neck:* No stiffness, pain, or swelling

4. *Endocrine:* No hot/cold intolerance, polyuria, or polydipsia

5. *Hematologic:* No trouble with bleeding or bruising. Never told of anemia

6. *Lymph nodes:* None enlarged

7. *Lungs:* No SOB, sputum, cough, night sweats, or TB exposure

8. *CV:* No CP, palpitations, syanosis, orthopnea, or PND

9. *GI:* Good appetite. No indigestion, heartburn, N&V, diarrhea, constipation, PUD, blood, or black stools

10. *GU:* No dysuria, frequency, hesitancy, or H/O UTIs

11. *NM:* No weakness, seizures, numbness, or tremor

12. *General:* No fever, chills, or weight change

G. PHYSICAL EXAM

P = 80 regular supine, 84 standing; BP = 150/95 supine; RR = 16 unlabored; Ht = 5'10"; Wt = 242 lb; Temp = 37.9C (oral)

1. *General:* The patient is a moderately obese white male who cannot put any weight on his left leg. He is alert and oriented but in obvious discomfort

2. *Skin:* Mild erythema over left knee. Several actinic keratoses on face and forearms. No other rashes, petechiae, splinters, or pustules

3. *Skeletal:* Left knee has moderate-sized effusion and is warm. Any movement of the knee causes pain. Otherwise all joints have full ROM and no effusions or synovitis. No tophi

4. *Head:* NC/AT

5. *Eyes:* Sclerae and conjuctivae clear; visual fields full to confrontation; EOM full and smooth; PERRLA; fundi show flat disks with no sign of papilledema. Mild arteriolar narrowing

6. *Ears:* Hearing normal to watch tick; Rinne's a > b; Weber's midline; TMs normal

7. *Nose:* Septum midline; no discharge

8. *Mouth and throat:* No ulcers or other lesions; several dental caries

9. *Neck:* Supple without masses; thryoid not enlarged; no nodules

10. *LN:* No cervical, axillary, supraclavicular, or inguinal lymphadenopathy

11. *Lungs:* Full inspiratory motion; no fremitus; clear to PA

12. *CV:* No JVD; PMI at 5th ICS at MCL; no thrills or heaves; normal S_1 and S_2; no S_3 or S_4. I-II/VI SEM at LLSB without radiation; no diastolic murmur or rubs

13. *Pulses:* Radial, brachial, femoral, DP, PT all full and symmetrical without bruits

14. *Abdomen:* Moderately obese; BS no; no bruit; liver percusses to 8 cm and lower border palpable at RCM; no palpable spleen, masses, or aorta; no tenderness or guarding

15. *GU:* N1 (normal) male; no testicular masses; no discharge

16. *Rectal:* 2+ prostate; no masses or tenderness; stool brown; guaiac negative

17. Neurologic
    a. *MS:* Alert, 0 x 3
    b. *CV:* II-XII intact
    c. *Motor:* All muscles 5/5 (left leg not tested)
    d. *Sensory:* Intact to light touch, vibration, pinprick, proprioception
    e. *Cerebellar:* H→S normal; RAM normal; F→N normal
    f. *DTRs:* All 2+ (left knee not tested). Toes downgoing

18. Labs
    a. *CBC:* Hct = 44; WBC = 24,500 (80PMN, 14 bands, 6 lymphs); platelets 244,000
    b. *Chem:* $\dfrac{140}{4.1} \Big| \dfrac{99}{25} \Big| \dfrac{14}{141} \Big\backslash 0.9$
    c. *Urine:* Clear yellow; sg 1.020; ph = 6; prot −; SSA −; gluc −; ket −; no cells or casts seen
    d. *CXR:* Normal
    e. *ECG:* NSR, rate = 76; no acute changes
    f. *Synovial fluid (from ER):* 70,000 WBC (98% PMN); 150 RBC; Gram's stain = no organisms
    g. *Knee x-ray (from ER):* Effusion, no bony abnormalities

H. ASSESSMENT AND PLANS

1. Assessment
    a. *Acute monoarthritis of left knee:* This patient presents with a 1-day history of severe pain and swelling of the knee. On exam he has a low-grade fever and his labs show a leukocytosis with left shift. The knee fluid was very inflammatory. The major diagnostic possibilities follow
        (1) *Septic joint:* His entire presentation is consistent with this diagnosis. A positive Gram's stain would have been diagnostic. If sepsis, staph and strep

would be the most likely bacteria. GC also needs to be considered, but his age, and the lack of skin symptoms, other joint symptoms, or discharge would argue against this diagnosis. Atypical infections such as TB or fungus would be unusual in an otherwise healthy man. Treatment for a bacterial pyarthrosis consists of drainage and antibiotics

(2) *Gout (or pseudogout):* He is at risk for gout because of his sex, obesity, hypertension, and drinking. His previous history of "gout" is of interest. Gout could certainly cause the severe degree of pain and fever. Unfortunately, a crystal exam was not performed on the synovial fluid obtained in the ER. The presence of crystals would not R/O infection

(3) *Trauma:* No history. X-ray shows nothing. High degree of inflammation not typical

(4) *Spondyloarthropathy, such as Reiter's syndrome:* No other findings to suggest this (eye inflammation, rash, or discharge), but could cause severe monoarthritis

(5) *RA:* Would be unusual presentation

b. *Hypertension (HTN):* No suggestion by electrolytes, urinalysis, or physical exam that his HTN is anything but essential hypertension. For now will observe BP in hospital. If he has gout, a diuretic might worsen it

c. *H/O alcohol abuse:* Apparently not a problem now, but will observe for signs of withdrawal

d. *Drug intolerance:* Nausea with codeine

e. *S/P appendectomy*

f. *Systolic ejection murmur:* Probably physiologic

Overall, infection and gout are most likely.

2. *Plans*

a. Frequent aspiration of the knee with large gauge needle (tap dry)

b. Examination of synovial fluid for crystals. If positive, treat patient for gout

c. Blood cultures now and for any fever

d. Keep flow sheet of fluid volumes and cell counts

e. Orthopedics consult for possible surgical drainage of knee

f. Synovial fluid cultures pending

g. Darvon for pain (will not suppress fever)

h. Bedrest for now

i. Start antibiotics with nafcillin and gentamicin

Appendix II. Sample Case Presentation

Mr. _____ is a 53-year-old married, white, bricklayer admitted for management of an acute pyarthrosis of the left knee.

He has generally been healthy except for mild hypertension—treated intermittently with HCTZ—and a distant history of alcohol abuse. His present illness began yesterday morning. He woke with pain and swelling of the left knee that progressed over the course of the day. He finally presented to the ER in the early afternoon complaining that his knee pain was the worst pain that he had ever had. In the ER he was found to have a fever of 38.4C and aspiration of the knee produced 60 cc of cloudy fluid with 70,000 WBC, 98% PMNs. Cultures were sent, but the fluid was not examined for crystals. Therefore, he was admitted to rule out a septic knee. He denied any history of gout, podagra, fevers, chills, trauma, pain elsewhere, rashes, discharge, or family history of gout, or arthritis.

The past medical history, family history, social history, and review of systems were otherwise noncontributory.

On exam, the patient was a moderately obese white man alert and oriented, but in obvious discomfort from knee pain. Pulse was 80 and blood pressure 150/95 without orthostatic change. Temperature was 37.9C and respiratory rate 16. Skin exam showed no focal lesions although there was erythema around the left knee. The knee itself had a large effusion present and was warm and very tender. Any movement of the knee caused a lot of pain. Other joints were normal and no tophi were seen. HEENT exam was unremarkable except for mild arteriolar narrowing. Lungs were clear. Cardiovascular exam showed a grade I-II/VI systolic

125

ejection murmur at the lower left sternal border, but was otherwise normal. Abdominal exam showed a normal-sized liver, no palpable masses or spleen.

The remainder of the physical exam, including neurologic exam, was unremarkable.

Laboratory data included a hematocrit of 44, WBC count of 24,500 with 80% PMNs and 14% bands. Electrolytes, urinalysis, chest x-ray and ECG were normal. X-ray of the left knee was normal except for the presence of an effusion.

In summary, this is a previously healthy man presenting with an acute pyarthrosis of the left knee.

Appendix III. Sample Admission Orders

5-25-88
6 P.M.

1. Admit to 6113, Dr. Ramone

2. *Diagnosis:* Pyarthrosis of knee

3. *Condition:* Fair

4. *Allergies:* Codeine (nausea)

5. *VS:* q4h

6. *Activity:* Bedrest

7. *Diet:* Regular

8. IV team to start and maintain heplock

9. *Medications:* Nafcillin 2 g IV q4h; gentamicin 120 mg IV now, then 80 mg IV q8h; Darvon 65 mg p.o. q4h p.r.n. pain; MOM 30 cc p.o. p.r.n. constipation

10. *Labs:* CBC and differential—A.M. draw tomorrow

11. Call HO for temp >38C; BP >160/100 or <120/80; P >120 or <60

12. ECG tonight

13. Chest x-ray tonight "Pyarthrosis of knee"

14. Orthopedics consult, Dr. Rotten, "Please evaluate patient with pyarthrosis of knee." He has been notified

Appendix IV. Common Abbreviations

AAA. Abdominal aortic aneurysm
A-a gradient. Alveolar arterial gradient
Ab. Antibiotic; antibody; abortion
ABG. Arterial blood gas
a.c. Before eating
ACBE. Air contrast barium enema
ad lib. Unrestricted
ADA. American Diabetes Association (diet)
AF. Atrial fibrillation; afebrile; aortofemoral
AFB. Acid-fast bacillus
AFP. Alpha-fetoprotein
AG. Anion gap
AI. Aortic insufficiency
AKA. Above the knee amputation
ALL. Acute lymphocytic leukemia
AML. Acute myelogenous leukemia
ANA. Antinuclear antibody (*see* FANA)
AODM. Adult onset diabetes mellitus
AP. Anteroposterior; abdominal–perineal
A&P. Assessment and plans
AR. Aortic regurgitation
ARDS. Adult respiratory distress syndrome
ARF. Acute renal failure; acute rheumatic failure
AS. Aortic stenosis
ASA. Aspirin
asap. As soon as possible
ASCVD. Atherosclerotic cardiovascular disease
ASD. Atrial septal defect
ASO. Antistreptolysin O

AV. Atrioventricular; arteriovenous
AVM. Arteriovenous malformation
A&W. Alive and well
AXR. Abdominal x-ray
B I&II. Billroth I&II
BBB. Bundle branch block (*see* RBBB, LBBB)
BE. Barium enema
b.i.d. Twice a day
BKA. Below the knee amputation
BM. Bone marrow; bowel movement
BP. Blood pressure
BPD. Biparietal diameter
BPH. Benign prostatic hypertrophy
BRBPR. Bright red blood per rectum
BRP. Bathroom privileges
BS. Bowel sounds; breath sounds
BS&O. Bilateral salpingo-oophorectomy
BUN. Blood urea nitrogen
Bx. Biopsy
c. With
Ca. Cancer; calcium
CABG. Coronary artery bypass graft
CT. Computerized tomography
CBC. Complete blood count
CC. Chief complaint
CCU. Clean-catch urine; coronary care unit
CEA. Carcinoembryonic antigen
CF. Cystic fibrosis
CGL. Chronic granulocytic leukemia
CHF. Congestive heart failure
CHO. Carbohydrate
CI. Cardiac index
CK. Creatine kinase
CML. Chronic myelogenous leukemia
CMV. Cytomegalovirus
CN. Cranial nerves
CNS. Central nervous system
CO. Cardiac output; carbon monoxide
c/o. Complaining of

COPD. Chronic obstructive pulmonary disease
CP. Chest pain; cerebral palsy
CPAP. Continuous positive airway pressure
CPC. Chronic passive congestion; clinical–pathological conference
CPK. Creatine phosphokinase
CPPD. Calcium pyrophosphate dihydrate (pseudogout)
CPR. Cardiopulmonary resuscitation
CrCl. Creatinine clearance
CRF. Chronic renal failure
CRP. C-reactive protein
C&S. Culture and sensitivity
CSF. Cerebrospinal fluid
CT. Computed tomography
CV. Cardiovascular; cerebrovascular
CVA. Cerebrovascular accident; costovertebral angle
CVP. Central venous pressure
c/w. Consistent with
Cx. Culture
CXR. Chest x-ray
DC. Discharge
D/C. Discontinue
D&C. Dilation and curettage
DDx. Differential diagnosis
DEA. Drug enforcement administration
DI. Diabetes insipidus
DIC. Disseminated intravascular coagulation
DIP. Distal interphalangeal joint
DJD. Degenerative joint disease
DKA. Diabetic ketoacidosis
DLE. Discoid lupus erythematosus
DM. Diabetes mellitus
DNR. Do not resuscitate
DOA. Dead on arrival
DOE. Dyspnea on exertion
DP. Dorsalis pedis
DPH. Diphenyl hydantoin (Dilantin)
DPT. Diphtheria-pertussis-tetanus
DSD. Dry sterile dressing
DT. Delirium tremens

DTR. Deep tendon reflex
DVT. Deep venous thrombosis
Dx. Diagnosis
EBL. Estimated blood loss
ECG. Electrocardiogram
ECT. Electroconvulsive therapy
EDC. Estimated date of confinement (due date)
EDTA. Ethylendiaminetetra acetic acid
EFM. External fetal monitor
EGA. Estimated gestational age
EMG. Electromyogram
ENT. Ear, nose, and throat
EOM. Extraocular muscles or movements
ER. Emergency room
ERCP. Endoscopic retrograde cholangiopancreatography
ESR. Erythrocyte sedimentation rate (*see* WESR)
ET. Endotrachial
ETOH. Ethanol
ETS. Endotracheal suction
ETT. Endotrachial tube; exercise treadmill test
EUA. Examination under anesthesia
FANA. Fluorescent ANA
FAT. Fetal activity test
FBS. Fasting blood sugar
FEV_1. Forced expiratory volume at 1 second
FFP. Fresh frozen plasma
FH. Family history; fundal height
FHT. Fetal heart tones
FLK. Funny looking kid
FOS. Full of stool
FRC. Functional residual capacity
FTA-ABS. Fluorescent trepanemal antibody-absorbed
FU. Follow-up
FUO. Fever of unknown origin
FVC. Forced vital capacity
Fx. Fracture
G. Gravida
GC. Gonorrhea
GCA. Gonococcal arthritis; giant cell arteritis

GGT. Gamma glutamyl transpeptidase
GFR. Glomerular filtration rate
GI. Gastrointestinal
GSW. Gunshot wound
gt, gtt. Drop; drops
GTT. Glucose tolerance test
GU. Genitourinary
GXT. Graded exercise tolerance
HA. Headache
HAA. Hepatitis associated antigen (HBsAg)
HBsAg. Hepatitis B surface antigen
HBP. High blood pressure
HCG. Human chorionic gonadotropin
Hct. Hematocrit
HCTZ. Hydrochlorothiazide
H&E. Hemorrhages and exudates; hematoxylin and eosin
HEENT. Head, eyes, ears, nose, and throat
Hgb. Hemoglobin
H/H. Hemoglobin/hematocrit
HJR. Hepatojugular reflux
HO. House officer
H/O. History of
HOB. Head of bed
H&P. History and physical
HPF. High-power field
HPI. History of present illness
HR. Heart rate
h.s. Bedtime
HSM. Hepatosplenomegaly
HSV. Herpes simplex virus
HTN. Hypertension
Hx. History
ICS. Intercostal space
ICU. Intensive care unit (*see* MICU, PICU, SICU, NICU)
ID. Infectious disease; identification
I&D. Incision and drainage
IDDM. Insulin dependent diabetes mellitus
Ig. Immunoglobulin
IHSS. Idiopathic hypertrophic subaortic stenosis

IJ. Internal jugular
IM. Intramuscular
IMV. Intermittent mandatory ventilation
INH. Isoniazid
I&O. Intake and output
IPPB. Intermittent positive pressure breathing
IT. Intrathecal
ITP. Idiopathic (immune) thrombocytopenic purpura
IUP. Intrauterine pregnancy
IV. Intravenous
IVC. Intravenous cholangiogram
IVP. Intravenous pyelogram
JAR. Junior Assistant Resident
JODM. Juvenile onset diabetes mellitus
JVD. Jugular venous distension
KUB. Kidneys, ureters, bladder (x-ray)
KVO. Keep vein open
L. Left
LAD. Left axis deviation; left anterior descending
LAE. Left atrial enlargement
LAHB. Left anterior hemiblock
LAP. Left atrial pressure
LBBB. Left bundle branch block
LE. Lupus erythematosis (*see* SLE, DLE)
LIH. Left inguinal hernia
LLL. Left lower lobe
LLSB. Lower left sternal border
LMD. Local medical doctor
LMP. Last menstrual period
LN. Lymph nodes
LOC. Loss of consciousness
LP. Lumbar puncture
LPN. Licensed practical nurse
LSB. Left sternal border
LUQ. Left upper quadrant
LV. Left ventricle
LVEDP. Left ventricular end-diastolic pressure
LVH. Left ventricular hypertrophy
MAP. Mean arterial pressure

MBT. Maternal blood type
MCH. Mean cell hemoglobin
MCHC. MCH concentration
MCL. Midclavicular line
MCP. Metacarpophalangeal (joint)
MCV. Mean cell volume
MI. Myocardial infarct; mitral insufficiency
MICU. Medical ICU
MMEF. Maximal midexpiratory flow
MMR. Measles, mumps, rubella (vaccine)
MR. Mitral regurgitation
MRI. Magnetic resonance imaging
MS. Mitral stenosis; morphine sulfate; multiple sclerosis; musculoskel-
    etal
MVA. Motor vehicle accident
MVI. Multivitamin
NAD. No active disease
NAS. No added salt
NC/AT. Normocephalic/atraumatic
NCV. Nerve conduction velocity
NG. Nasogastric
NICU. Neonatal ICU
NIDDM. Noninsulin dependent diabetes mellitus
NKA. No known allergies
NM. Neuromuscular
NPH. Neutral protamine Hagedorn (insulin); normal pressure hydro-
    cephalus
n.p.o. Nothing by mouth
NR. Nonreactive
NS. Normal saline; neurosurgery
NSAID. Nonsteroidal anti-inflammatory drug
NSR. Normal sinus rhythm
NT. Nasotrachial
NTG. Nitroglycerine
N&V. Nausea and vomiting
OA. Osteoarthritis
OB. Obstetrics
OCG. Oral cholecystogram
OCP. Oral contraceptive pills

OD. Overdose; right eye
OM. Otitis media
OOB. Out of bed
OOT. Out of town
OR. Operating room
OS. Left eye; opening snap
OT. Occipito-transverse
OTD. Out the door
OU. Both eyes
P. Pulse; para
PA. Pulmonary artery; physician's assistant; posteroanterior; pernicious
    anemia
PAC. Premature atrial contraction
PAP. Pulmonary artery pressure
PAT. Paroxysmal atrial tachycardia
PBC. Primary biliary cirrhosis
p.c. After eating
pcn. Penicillin
pcm. Penicillamine
PCWP. Pulmonary capillary wedge pressure
PDA. Patent ductus arteriosis
PDR. Physicians' Desk Reference
PE. Physical exam; pulmonary embolus
PEEP. Positive end-expiratory pressure
PERRLA. Pupils round, react to light, and accommodate
PFT. Pulmonary function tests
PICU. Pediatric ICU
PID. Pelvic inflammatory disease
PIP. Proximal interphalangeal (joint)
PMH. Past medical history
PMI. Point of maximal impulse
p MN. After midnight
PMN. Polymorphonuclear neutrophil
PND. Paroxysmal nocturnal dyspnea
p.o. By mouth
PP. Postpartum; pulsus paradoxus; postprandial
P&PD. Percussion and postural drainage
PPD. Purified protein derivative
PPN. Parenteral nutrition

p.r. Per rectum
PRBC. Packed red blood cells
p.r.n. As needed
PS. Pulmonic stenosis
PT. Prothrombin time; physical therapy; posterior tibial
pt. Patient
PTA. Prior to admission
PTCA. Percutaneous transluminal coronary angioplasty
PTH. Parathormone
PTHC. Percutaneous transhepatic cholangiography
PTT. Partial thromboplastin time
PUD. Peptic ulcer disease
PVC. Premature ventricular contraction
PVD. Peripheral vascular disease
q. Every
q.d. Every day
q.h. Every hour
q.h.s. Every bedtime
q.i.d. Four times a day
QNS. Quantity not sufficient
q.o.d. Every other day
R. Right; respirations
RA. Rheumatoid arthritis; right atrium
RAD. Right axis deviation
RAE. Right atrial enlargement
RBBB. Right bundle branch block
RBC. Red blood cell
RCM. Right costal margin
RF. Rheumatoid factor; rheumatic fever
RIA. Radioimmunoassay
RIH. Right inguinal hernia
RLL. Right lower lobe
RLQ. Right lower quadrant
RML. Right middle lobe
R/O. Rule out
ROA. Right occipito-anterior
ROM. Range of motion
ROP. Right occipito-posterior
ROS. Review of systems

ROT. Right occipito-transverse
RPR. Rapid plasma reagin
RPR-NR. Rapid plasma reagin-nonreactive
RR. Recovery room; respiratory rate
RRR. Regular rate and rhythm
RSB. Right sternal border
RT. Radiation therapy (rad Rx); respiratory therapy
RTA. Renal tubular acidosis
RTC. Return to clinic
RTO. Return to office
RUG. Retrograde urethrogram
RUL. Right upper lobe
RUQ. Right upper quadrant
RV. Residual volume
RVH. Right ventricular hypertrophy
Rx. Therapy
s. Without
SA. Sinoatrial
S&A. Sugar and acetone
SAR. Senior Assistant Resident
SBE. Subacute bacterial endocarditis
SBFT. Small bowel follow-through
SC. Service connected (VA)
SCM. Sternocleidomastoid
SEM. Systolic ejection murmur; standard error of the mean
SG. Swan–Ganz
sg. Specific gravity
SH. Social history
SIADH. Syndrome of inappropriate ADH
SICU. Surgical ICU
SKSD. Streptokinase streptodornase
SL. Sublingual
SLE. Systemic lupus erythematosus
SMA. Sequential multiple analysis
SOAP. Subjective, objective, assessment, plans
SOB. Shortness of breath
S/P. Status post
SQ. Subcutaneous
SROM. Spontaneous rupture of membranes

SSA. Sulfasalic acid
stat. Immediately
STS. Serologic test for syphilis
SVD. Spontaneous vaginal delivery
SVT. Supraventricular tachycardia
Sx. Symptoms
TAH. Total abdominal hysterectomy
TB. Tuberculosis
TBLC. Term birth living child
T&C. Type and cross
TC&DB. Turn, cough, and deep breathe
TED. Thromboembolic disease support (hose)
TFT. Thyroid function test
T&H. Type and hold
TIA. Transient ischemic attack
TIBC. Total iron binding capacity
t.i.d. Three times a day
TKO. To keep open
TLC. Tender loving care; total lung capacity
TM. Tympanic membrane; time
TMJ. Temporomandibular joint
TNTC. Too numerous to count
TOPV. Trivalent oral polio vaccine
TORCH. Toxoplasma, rubella, cytomegalovirus, herpes
TPN. Total parenteral nutrition
TPR. Temperature, pulse, and respirations
TR. Tricuspid regurgitation
TRU. T3 resin uptake
TTP. Thrombotic thrombocytopenic purpura
TU. Tuberculin units
TURP. Transurethral resection of the prostate
TV. Tidal volume
TVH. Total vaginal histerectomy
Tx. Treatment; transfer; transplant
U. Unit
UA. Urinalysis; uric acid
UCHD. Usual childhood diseases
UGI. Upper gastrointestinal
URI. Upper respiratory infection

U/S. Ultrasound
UTI. Urinary tract infection
VAH. Veterans' Administration Hospital
VDRL. Venereal disease research lab
V/Q. Ventilation perfusion
VS. Vital signs
VSS. Vital signs stable
WBC. White blood cell
WD. Well developed
WESR. Westegren ESR
WN. Well nourished
WNL. Within normal limits
X. Times
$\bar{x}$. Except
yo. Years old

NOTES

NOTES

NOTES

NOTES

NOTES

NOTES

NOTES

NOTES

NOTES

NOTES